A
Toughest Fight

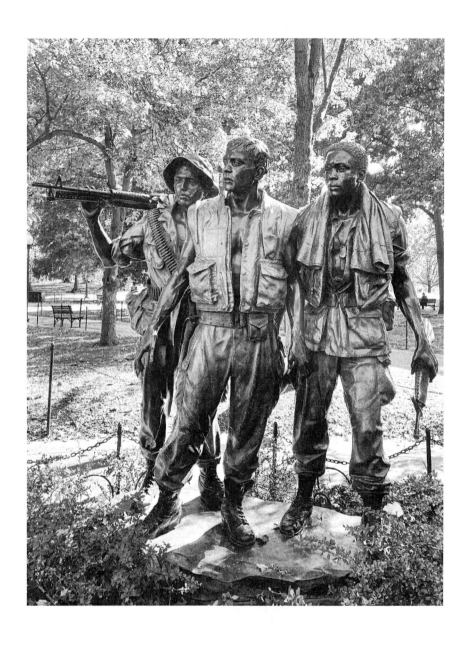

A Veteran's Toughest Fight

Finding Peace After Vietnam

David T. Klein

Foreword by Edward Tick

McFarland & Company, Inc., Publishers
Jefferson, North Carolina

Frontispiece: "Three Soldiers" bronze statue by Frederick Hart, Vietnam Memorial Wall in Washington, D.C.

LIBRARY OF CONGRESS CATALOGING-IN-PUBLICATION DATA

Names: Klein, David, 1968– author. | Tick, Edward, writer of foreword.
Title: A veteran's toughest fight : finding peace after Vietnam / David Klein ; foreword by Edward Tick.
Other titles: Finding peace after Vietnam
Description: Jefferson, North Carolina : McFarland & Company, Inc., Publishers, 2024 | Includes index.
Identifiers: LCCN 2024026030 | ISBN 9781476695419 (paperback : acid free paper) ∞
ISBN 9781476652856 (ebook)
Subjects: LCSH: Vietnam War, 1961-1975—Veterans—United States. | Vietnam War, 1961–1975—Anecdotes. | Vietnam War, 1961–1975—Veterans—Mental health—United States. | Veterans—United States—Social conditionns. | Veterans—Mental health—United States.
Classification: LCC DS559.73.U6 K54 2024 | DDC 959.704/340922—dc23
LC record available at https://lccn.loc.gov/2024026030

BRITISH LIBRARY CATALOGUING DATA ARE AVAILABLE

ISBN (print) 978-1-4766-9541-9
ISBN (ebook) 978-1-4766-5285-6

Front cover image: photograph of Marine on patrol at sunrise in I Corps, RVN (author collection)

Printed in the United States of America

McFarland & Company, Inc., Publishers
 Box 611, Jefferson, North Carolina 28640
 www.mcfarlandpub.com

To all of the U.S. military men and women who
deployed to Vietnam, the 58,220 who perished,
the many who have died since due to their service,
and the countless survivors who were
forever changed by the war.
It is especially dedicated to all of the veterans
with whom I have had the honor to serve in their
decades-long search for healing and recovery.

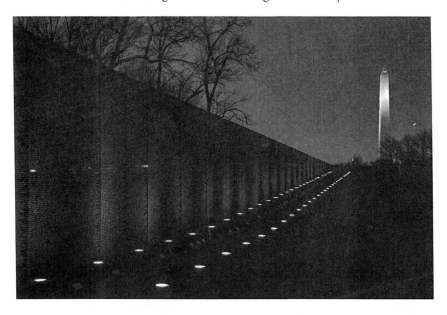

Vietnam War Memorial in Washington, D.C., at night. Wikimedia Commons.

Acknowledgments

I wish to thank so many who have supported the creation and publication of this book. My immediate family and friends who offered their love, confidence, and support are numerous, and are indispensable in my life and my work. Thank you for the countless hours of reading, editing, opining, and loving me through this process. Your investments in me are too many to list. I am the person, professional, and author I am because of my connections with you. I love you all. I trust you know who you are.

I would also like to express gratitude to a small group of professionals that directly assisted this book to life. That group includes Drs. Edward Tick, Zachary Shore, and Jennifer King who have contributed to the ideas, editing, development, mentorship and friendship that helped honed my ideas, writing and book structure.

I would also like to thank Charlie Perdue, Acquisitions Editor, and his team at McFarland & Company, for giving me and this book a chance, and for the facility and spirit in which they have guided the process from submission to publication.

Finally, while I have dedicated this book to them, I wish to acknowledge all of the veterans who have personally let me into their worlds and have also provided me the opportunity to travel alongside of them for their healing journey, and for all they have taught me about resilience, trauma, life, death, war, and peace. Perhaps most of all, they have held up the largest of mirrors and gifted me the chance to learn about myself, to become a better psychologist and healer, and a better American citizen and person.

Table of Contents

II—Transformation and Return   125

Foreword
by Edward Tick

The tales of King Arthur and his Knights of the Round Table are some of Western Civilization's core heroic myths. Myths are not just entertainment, literature, or cultural artifacts. Myths are guides for the soul for our deepest life journeys. They are archetypal patterns that replicate time and again throughout human history. Myths are stories we all live in their contemporary versions.

The 2021 movie *The Green Knight* is a cinematic retelling of the Arthurian legend of "Sir Gawain and the Green Knight." In the movie version, an aging King Arthur calls his nephew young Gawain to stand before the throne and says, "Tell me your story that I may know you." Gawain, not yet a knight, shyly admits he does not yet have a story. The tale unfolds as the uninitiated, untested young squire lives his strange, demanding, life-threatening journey that tests him to the utmost and transforms him so that it becomes his initiation into manhood and knighthood.

Without our stories that expose us to life's naked truths and test our characters before ultimate matters, we do not mature to become adults or knights, that is, true warriors.

When Dr. Klein was young David, he knew he wanted to write. As he tells us herein, he was a war baby, born during the Viet Nam War and in an almost mystical way bonded to its veterans his entire life. But he did not yet have his story, so he did not write his book. His fascination with, attraction to, and lifelong service as psychotherapist to Viet Nam War veterans became his mythic journey and his initiation, ultimately, into their brotherhood, his purpose as a writer, and his own inner warriorhood. *A Veteran's Toughest Fight* is evidence of that sacred journey—in service to our veterans and to his own soul as well.

War has been ubiquitous in the human experience. There have been at least 15,000 wars in the last 5,000 years of recorded history and to this day.

And so, the trauma and suffering caused by war has also been omnipresent in human history. There have been many ways throughout the millennia of conceiving war's invisible wounds that today we call Post-Traumatic Stress Disorder and Moral Injury; we know of more than eighty names these have been given through the ages and cultures. Conceiving of it as a pathology is only our modern quasi-scientific version. One contrasting example of many is the Lakota (Sioux) conception of the wound. In their language it is known as "the spirits left." In traditional cultures it is conceived as a spiritual wound, a deep wound to the soul, and its remedy, therefore, is restoring the spirit of the depleted warrior.

Warriors have their horrific ordeals and need their stories. Story is critical to warrior healing and restoration. To restore the warrior's spirit, we must support her or him in "re-storying." To disallow storytelling, as well-intentioned brief therapies do, is to betray the warrior by blocking necessary steps in their healing and homecoming. This is often done for fear of "retraumatizing." One Viet Nam War nurse told me, after completing a residential treatment program for PTSD, "They only allowed one short afternoon for storytelling. I was not allowed to tell my stories. I don't feel healed; I feel lobotomized."

Thus, one healing formula for our veterans can be: To restore, re-story. Telling the story recreates psychic order in the inner world that had become fragmented and disordered during warfare and its inevitable traumas. In this effort, Dr. Klein is supreme. This book demonstrates the wisdom, power, methodology, and potentially transformative power of "restorying to restore."

There are several critical phases of the warrior's return journey. I have presented the six "Necessities of Return" in my work and books *War and the Soul* and *Warrior's Return*. These are isolation and tending, purification and cleansing, affirmation of destiny, storytelling, restitution, and finally, initiation. Though Dr. Klein—David's—book concentrates on storytelling, all the elements of warrior return are in fact present in his work and this volume.

Dr. Klein has served for decades as a Veterans Administration psychologist conducting countless individual and group therapy sessions for veterans; that is isolation and tending in safety and trust. His veterans come out of their closets as who they are and with what they did, recognized in their small and safe community of other vets—affirmation of destiny. They practice storytelling and deep and compassionate listening to each other as Dr. Klein facilitates. Through tears and the expression of buried memories and emotions, they achieve purification and cleansing. And sometimes, blessedly, as some of these stories testify, between each other, in their families, in society, and even in Viet Nam, they practice acts of witnessing, forgiveness, charity, giving back, and redemption that put their souls back to right order with all of life. This process, finally, brings restoration. It brings the warrior spirit back to the veteran who had been emptied of soul and thereby brings true warrior initiation.

But these stories and this initiation process are not just for the veterans. Dr. Klein courageously, skillfully, devotedly, empathically facilitates. This is also David's story. He was a young man fascinated with war, the military, veterans, but he did not serve and did not have his own story. His hero's journey became creating, guiding, facilitating, and writing the journeys of soul-wounded warriors so that their stories became his and their journeys his journey. What they could not speak, he enabled them to speak. What was horrendous and forbidden, he allowed to surface from the dark depths into the light. What civilians, as he says, out of either fear or ignorance could not listen to or tolerate, he, as he puts it, "fell in." He allowed himself to hear, see, smell, feel with his veterans. He took their imaginal journeys through the inner war zone as they had taken it in the hell of combat. Thus, David took the inner mythic journey as he led his veterans on the healing path.

Further, as I needed to long ago after my own decades of work with veterans, both his identities, David, and Dr. Klein, needed to make the pilgrimage to Viet Nam. The war had been in my imagination for decades when I first began leading annual healing journeys to that land in 2000; those twenty years are recorded in poetry in my volume *Coming Home in Viet Nam*. David and I took the journey together in 2016, for, as with veterans, it is necessary to see, hear, smell, feel that land, to know the real people and culture against which we waged war, to discover who they really are, how they have healed and moved on, and to replace the images of horror and suffering burnt into the mind that is at the core of the traumatic wound with the green, growing, happy, healthy, forgiving and loving people of Viet Nam as they are today.

Beyond that, David accepted the additional task of returning to that land some of his veterans' relics, memories, and messages for those who could not make the journey. He traveled in proxy for the numerous veterans he has helped heal. He traveled for reconciliation, understanding, and forgiveness for and from the Vietnamese. And he traveled for his own soul's journey to maturity and completion.

All this and more are in these stories that David has painstakingly and skillfully presented—and he is a good writer!—to us, to our country still in need of healing from that and our many wars, still in need of reconciliation and healing between our warrior and civilian classes. We must become one. This work helps achieve the critical goal of "communalization."

Communalization was first named as an essential component in veteran healing by Jonathan Shay in *Achilles in Vietnam*. There he describes it as "being able to safely tell the story to someone who is listening and who can be trusted to retell it truthfully to others in the community." In *Herakles Gone Mad*, Robert Emmet Meagher says the process "requires a live audience... able to feel each other's presence and see each other's pain.... This means mutual recognition and commitment." For all these reasons and more, I recast PTSD as Post-Traumatic Soul Distress and Post-Traumatic Social Disorder. As a non-veteran, listener, and storyteller, Dr. Klein is preeminent in providing that audience and communicating the stories to our society. As he succinctly declares, "without partnering in truth, there is no healing."

In this process, Dr. David Klein not only performed invaluable service that he could not have provided otherwise. He also entered the ancient sacred brotherhood and gained "priceless education and relationships." By reading this book, all of us, and our country, may also gain these necessary transformational boons.

Edward Tick, Ph.D., is a pioneering psychotherapist in healing war's invisible wounds. He has been working with Vietnam War veterans since the 1970s, leading journeys to Vietnam since 2000, and works with younger American and international veterans. He is author of the War and the Soul *and* Warrior's Return, *along with numerous other books and articles.*

Preface

A reflective silence filled the group therapy room. Joseph was the first to break it. He served as an Army Ranger and team leader of a Special Forces recon unit in Vietnam. He began to tell his story, opened his heart, and we all fell in.

His devotion came first—in spite of everything, he would do it all again. And it was more than most could imagine.

Too many times, he came as close to dying as a man could get. His luck nearly ran out the night his team was overrun by the enemy horde on that tiny firebase deep in the Vietnamese jungle. Their magazines were nearly

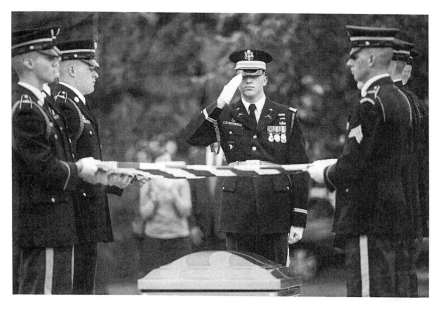

The ultimate sacrifice, Arlington National Cemetery, U.S. Army photograph, 18277112194, Larue.

empty when the shooting stopped. At daybreak, lifeless, contorted piles littered the smoldering perimeter. But they were alive. He didn't relish the killing, but it was easier once a man got used to the idea. Those memories were hard, but that wasn't the problem. There was only a single regret—one.

Joseph paused, his lip quivering, as he related why he couldn't let go of the war. He promised Will when it was all over, they would come home together. He was the team leader, but it was done before anyone could stop it. The day it happened, the American bullet that ended Will's life also killed something in him. Years in therapy passed before Joseph could tell this story aloud. He couldn't find the words to capture his pain or what he had lost in himself since that day.

After his tour, he returned the same way he arrived—alone. But home didn't feel like he remembered. In the jungle, the war silently pruned away the life he left behind. The hurt came in layers. Everyone back home lived as if nothing had changed. For him, nothing was the same. He tried to move on. He told himself the war was over. It wasn't.

Nights were the worst. Will visited him in the dark, pressing into Joseph's hidden ache. At first, the nightmares replayed that awful September day in a merciless loop. Then his mind wrestled with every variation that might undo Will's fate, but the truth refused to budge. After years of trauma work, the dreams shifted again, grasping for resolution.

Joseph wakes to the sound of running water. It draws him out of bed through a steamy dreamscape to the bathroom. There, he finds a youthful Will standing in the shower in his soaked jungle utilities. A warm gaze breaks into his boyish grin before offering assurances that he is okay as he washes the dark crimson stain from his right chest pocket.

But it wasn't okay.

Joseph's greatest anguish was it didn't seem to matter to anyone else, other than those who served, those who lost a son, brother, husband or father over there, or the minority of the American public who found a reason to care. Not mattering hurt. To those to whom it might, they couldn't possibly understand. For decades, he felt utterly alone.

But he wasn't now. He sat surrounded by reverent silence. The silence of men who were there and knew. The grief. The loneliness. The pain.

He ended this story to his trauma group with his deepest desire. Tears slowly followed the lines etched into his face by years of sorrow.

"I just wish my country loved and appreciated me as much as I love and appreciate it."

⌒

This book's aim is to unify our warrior storytellers and civilian listeners in healing. War creates pain—a pain that all of those who are touched by it, combatants and civilians alike, can, and often do, carry in some form for the rest of their lives. Joseph's story speaks for his generation of war veterans and to the largely disconnected civilian public. It conveys the agony of the isolated—people seeking connection and healing from war but not knowing how. They exist in parallel vexed by the problem of finding their way towards one another and yet, most of the time, those lines do not cross. This path of mutual isolation, I have found, is common among both veterans and those who care about them. Veterans need to tell their stories and we need to hear them.

Veterans deserve our appreciation for their service and to be healed of the wounds they incurred on our behalf. Civilians need to learn from their war experiences and value the hard-fought wisdom for which they paid so dearly. However, most of the time, this important exchange does not happen. So how do we bridge this division?

We do so through communalization and the sharing of story. This sacred process of returning from war and sharing ones' experiences with a nonjudgmental and empathic community of listeners, is not only helpful for them and us—it is essential; pain shared is pain divided. This timeless ritual has been performed across traditional, communal cultures since antiquity, but became lost as the social interconnectivity of our modern culture atrophied. The process of successful communalization emotionally and spiritually reconnects veterans to the rest of "us"—to their families, friends, and communities who sent them to war in our names. In turn, *they* and *us* become "we."

With ever fewer of us serving in the military on behalf of a growing and increasingly disconnected civilian majority, it is more important than ever to find our way towards one another. When our country offers its sons and daughters to war, we are all responsible for sharing the burden our warriors carry home with them. Those who are scarred by war demand our full attention and yet, most of the time, we conspire in silent avoidance. We don't ask, and they don't tell.

Most of what gets in the way can be reduced to one word—fear. They struggle to tell their story and we rarely know how to hear it. Therefore, veterans typically construct two versions of their service narratives—the safe story destined for public consumption and the *real* one. It spares both parties from the gamble.

We, civilians and veterans, are often scared of the same things; we are fearful of strong feelings, of judgment, of pain, and of seeing the human shadow we all carry inside of us. The veteran may suffer from moral injuries they wish to keep hidden. Simultaneously, the unscathed among us avert our eyes; we are scared to see what can become of every one of us when exposed to the human ugliness revealed when we wage war.

Ignorance also gets in the way. We may not know what to say or how to ask about a veteran's combat deployment. We may ask the wrong questions even when trying to convey genuine interest, or perhaps ask those same questions out of self-serving morbid curiosity. Too many veterans are asked how many people they killed, having little appreciation for the gravity of the question, and even less for the answer. Many veterans are asked sincere questions but are not offered the safety, space, respect, and compassion to answer them fully and honestly.

Sharing the stark reality of war's killing and destruction is an act of intimacy and, as such, a profound emotional risk. It is not the story most people want to hear, nor are many prepared or capable of hearing it. To open one's civilian ears and heart without judgment to the horrors of war also carries potential hazards. This, too, is part of what veterans fear—that the truth will offend, contaminate, or damage the unprepared listener.

Thus, rather than risk it, many veterans carry their burdens in lonely silence, still fulfilling their duties to protect their country's citizens at their own expense. This conspiracy of avoidance prevents the veteran and their communities from truly bringing our warriors home, learning from the experience of going to war, and healing our country's collective wounds. For all these reasons and more, the pain of war hides in darkness.

We need to witness these stories to emotionally tend to our warriors' health and well-being, and our civilian society is elemental to that process. This responsibility has, for too long, been delegated to the Department of Veterans Affairs, select mental health professionals, and clergy. While these healers help untold numbers of veterans, they cannot do this alone. Thus, community involvement and the communalization of combat experiences does not supplant formal treatment for PTSD and adjacent traumatic injuries—it complements it.

This compartmentalization of responsibility perpetuates our separation and thus the suffering of all involved. We need to be engaged from start to finish; veterans require our blessings when they deploy and require our partnership, honor, and support to "come home." Thanking our veterans for their service is a nice gesture, but that is not enough. They need us to be present and to listen. They deserve our commitment to them just as they committed to us, and sealed that compact with their bodies, their minds, and their lives. Our participation is not optional.

⁓

I devoted the majority of my career as a clinical psychologist to caring for and treating Vietnam combat veterans. For those who fought in that war, what they wanted most from their fellow Americans was the respectful understanding they earned with their sacrifice. Part of their collective pain is they were denied that dignity when they returned and that, to this day, so few people understand them.

Because of this rupture, so many coming back after the war never had a "home" to return to. Though over fifty years later, my hope is that their stories will contribute something towards the appreciation and honor they both earned and deserve.

This book is a collection of stories I witnessed in twenty-six years of clinical practice, and the priceless education and relationships that accompanied them. These stories are presented in an order that loosely traces the archetypal hero's journey. The first half of the book, *The Descent*, shares stories of these veterans' departure to Vietnam and their stark initiation into the ordeal of combat, facing the resulting trauma in treatment, or both. Its aim is to provide you with intimate portraits of the human costs of war. Sadly, some stories tell of those lost along the way in their attempts to reconcile those experiences. The second half, *Transformation and Return*, traces their journey home as changed men vying with their war experiences while they engage in the hard, but rewarding work of the trauma recovery process. It reveals typically private therapeutic exchanges, in both trauma-focused individual and group psychotherapy, and shares some of the methods that helped them find relief. Some of these veterans make appearances in more than one story and invite you to witness various angles and stages of their healing journey.

Some of the photographs that supplement this journey purposely avoid captions and, in so doing, are employed in a different fashion than most non-fiction books. I have assembled a variety of pictures including public domain combat photography from the Vietnam War; personal photographs of mine and my veterans (with permissions); and an assortment of stock and staged images that visually capture the essence of the story, pique your curiosity, and set an emotional tone without disclosing the storyline, thus preserving narrative tension. They invite some degree of your own projection or association to the picture. If those aims succeed, upon the story's completion, the lingering mental image symbolizes the story while enhancing your contemplation of what you just read.

These stories are shared with you to honor the unique experiences of these Vietnam veterans. Their selection was based on those that made profound impressions among the thousands of important stories I have witnessed over my career. While these stories are not intended to generalize to veterans of other wars, they tap and express a universality of the American warrior ordeal. Given the large numbers of those who served in Iraq, Afghanistan, and other combat theaters in the American Global War on Terror over the past two decades, the lessons learned from our Vietnam veterans, and our successes and mistakes in caring for them, are especially relevant right now.

Neither are these stories engineered with any predetermined themes or lessons in mind. They were written to capture biographical truths and the provocative experiences of suffering and triumph in response to combat. Some of these stories speak to the burden of living and dying with the aftermath of war. Some illuminate the hope and hard work of trauma recovery. Whether tragic or triumphant, it is their powerful and intimate authenticity that aims to connect us.

In so doing, these stories portray both the soaring human spirit and the treachery of men in combat. Yet their intentions are neither hawkish nor dovish with respect to war itself. If they are either or both, it is because these tales of survival organically speak to the full range of humanity found in the act of war and adaptation to its lasting impact. Finally, if these stories instruct us, it is because they speak to a raw truth and dark wisdom rarely found outside of the human tragedy of warfare.

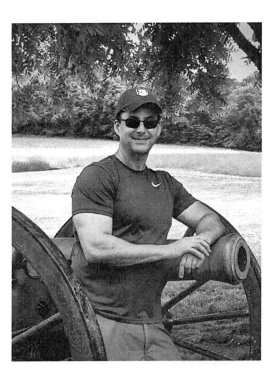

Sharing a trauma story is a profound act of courage and trust. Every effort has been made to morally, ethically, and legally honor that act.

This book consists of sensitive information on several levels. This is necessary because the aim is to confide real stories of war and its effects on those who have endured its legacy. Simultaneously, it pulls back the curtain on the protective secrecy created by the therapeutic encounter to promote understanding of veterans' trauma recovery process.

In order to honor these objectives, this book strives for a balance of authenticity and privacy.

The author at Wilson's Creek National (Civil War) Battlefield, Republic, MO.

These stories came to light in the context of confidential psychotherapeutic work. As a trauma psychologist, I have a privileged relationship with the veterans whose stories created this book. The word "privilege" here dually represents the ethical and legal duty to protect their privacy, as well as sincere appreciation of their trust, immersion in their unique worlds, and the gift of our relationship.

To honor privacy, personal identities have been changed, and reasonable efforts made to protect sensitive information. However, to honor the painful truth of those experiences and the memories of men they personally knew who died, where approved by the storyteller, actual names of the deceased are used. The intent is to honor those warriors' sacrifices and the memories of those who fought alongside them in combat. Pseudonyms for these heroes didn't feel right or meet that standard. Similarly, actual names/designations of larger military units, areas of operation, and physical locations were preserved in the service of historical accuracy where deemed to reasonably maintain confidentiality.

These necessary adjustments notwithstanding, the stories in this book are authentic. They are true as conveyed to me by the veteran based on memories of their war-related experiences in the context of their psychotherapy for the resulting trauma. While the serendipity, seeming coincidences, or events in some stories may test bounds of credibility, these stories were collected from trustworthy men of character and vetted wherever possible with collateral publicly available historical information. Accordingly, all stories are based on actual events, locations, and people. In my narration of these experiences, some limited creative license is employed to improve story flow, capture internal experiences of these veterans, and to promote understanding of their psychological experience of struggling with combat-related PTSD.

Because these stories are authentic, you may find some of their endings frustrating. The reality is that treatment of psychological trauma has its limits; in spite of advanced therapies, more effective medications and skilled practitioners, many treated trauma patients continue to struggle with refractory symptoms, moral injury, and functional impairments. Accordingly, some stories deny us Hollywood endings and comforting resolutions.

Informed written consent was granted for the use and publication of every story. These veterans were also given the opportunity to review the stories about them, offer edits on historical details, to approve or deny their inclusion in this book and to determine where use of pseudonyms could, when outside of a formal clinical relationship with myself, be waived. Where the subject of the story is deceased, next of kin provided consent.

These conditions were employed to achieve the goal of this book: that is, to create an honest compact in order to bring the story owner and his listener together. As I have argued, this union is essential in the communalization process—without partnering in truth, there is no healing.

⌒

I hope these stories inspire you as they have me. My aim is to engage fellow Americans in the challenges and joys of being present and listening to our veterans' stories with open hearts. While listening is therapeutic, it is not treatment, so one need not be a trained psychotherapist to do so. However, I intend to use my unique role as one to bring other civilians into the Vietnam combat veteran experience through their stories.

You may be a veteran, love and care about a veteran or, even in the absence of a personal connection, simply discover why their experiences should matter to us all. Also, like me, you may find yourself connected to Vietnam or other wars in ways you may not have anticipated. Upon reflection over my career—indeed, my life—that is precisely what I found when it mattered enough to begin looking.

Introduction

"I wasn't in country that long. We were on a chopper descending into the AO at Phu Hiep-2."

As they made their approach, the Lieutenant briefed the squad on the situation on the ground. The officer shouted over the deafening whirl of the rotors as the pilots accelerated them to flare the Huey and cushion their touchdown.

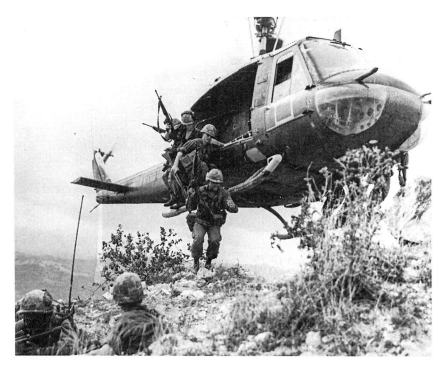

Helicopter insertion, U.S. Army photograph, U.S. Army SGT Howard Breedlove.

"The LZ isn't hot but be advised … they are interrogating prisoners."

Jack's shifting intonation signaled that we were beginning the descent into his nightmare. Tears began to spill over and run down his stubbled cheeks. His voice quivered, but his eyes remained locked with mine.

I felt my insides, without any conscious instruction, tighten in a guarding response, and yet I could not have felt more fully present. My mind spoke without guiding my lips to form the words.

"It's OK. I'm here and I'm going in there with you."

His eyes dropped, and he continued to speak.

"My squad set up on one side of the village. Then I saw them. The 'prisoners' the Lieutenant had talked about … were a mother and her two children. There were some South Vietnamese military security services and some CIA conducting the interrogations. I couldn't believe what I was seeing. They had a rag in the mother's mouth—they were waterboarding her in front of her kids…"

The wailing children hugged one another as they watched in helpless horror as the person who protected them most from this treacherous world choked and gagged on the steady stream of the village's well water.

Jack turned to the soldier next to him, half-pleading, half-hoping that this ally could somehow make what he was being forced to witness stop.

"We *can't* do this. We can't do *this*…," Jack cried.

The teenage soldier he looked to for some mercy had been there many months—a virtual lifetime for an infantryman in Vietnam. Whatever moral flame he brought with him into the war had already extinguished into a wispy ribbon of smoke in the service of what was necessary to survive.

"It's none of our business. If you can't look, go on the other side of that tree."

It was unclear if those words were meant to assure Jack, chastise him, or exculpate them both.

Jack's sense of time that day was obliterated by the show of inhumanity in front of him. I could see the frozen horror in his eyes as he continued to darken the scene with what the interrogators did next. If it were possible, and it had to be to honor the raw truth of what he witnessed, the details of that story opened into yet another deeper cavern of cruelty and depravity…

⁓

Everyone wants to do something that matters. Since the beginning of my career, I was told I should write a book. Early on, I believed one might naturally emerge as a byproduct of my years of work as a clinical psychologist in a combat trauma recovery program at a VA medical center. However, my mission was clinical work and becoming an author was not my priority. Even so, I never ruled it out as something that may come in time. Get enough experience, become an expert, write a book. Seemed logical enough.

So, I set about becoming that expert, not to write, but in an effort to help the hundreds of veterans I saw seeking relief from the emotional war injuries they carried. Though they were my primary teachers, I studied a lot such that I might eventually learn enough to really make a difference. Along the way, I collected information on trauma work that interested me and helped me help them.

In my many office files is one with the mundane tab labeled "writing." It is stuffed with a menagerie of quotes, articles, various snippets of trauma-relevant literature, and an occasional burst of intellectual inspiration that I experienced, jotted down and tossed in this file. Over time, that file continued to fatten but didn't coalesce into anything resembling a literary plan; the dormant book sat inside me for years, idling.

I told myself I was simply too busy to write it. However, the truth was that I was scared. I was scared to create something unoriginal that added nothing to our understanding of the subjective experience of combat veterans in general, and Vietnam veterans in particular. Beneath that layer was the deeper fear that I didn't know enough and was not worthy of being the voice behind these warriors' sacred stories. Most of all, I was scared if I tried, I would let them down.

Anything worth writing would have to honor them, their sacrifices for our country, and all that they have taught me. That was a tall order and, frankly, not one I was sure I could fill.

While I've worked in varying degrees with veterans of many wars, my visceral and spiritual connection was always with Vietnam veterans. I felt this connection as long as I can remember—they were "my guys"—always have been. Early on, I was not sure why. Nor did I fully grasp what I would encounter when I came to know them and why they became my life's mission. Now I know.

I have led over 5,000 PTSD group sessions for Vietnam combat veterans. I also spent countless hours over the course of my career providing individual therapy for them. I've listened to their stories for the last twenty-six years. I want to share some of those stories with you and hope they have the profound impact I discovered.

What I couldn't fathom when I started my work with these veterans was that I was not there just to heal and transform them; they were also going to transform me. I was on my own hero's journey and didn't know it. Upon my introduction to these warriors, I started the descent into my own ordeal. And while I thought my role was to guide them through the dark underworld, they were, simultaneously, guiding me.

To accompany them there, I had to leave my civilian world, one cloaked in safety and comfort. I needed to follow them through the gauntlet of war—the experience that irreparably altered their lives. No one makes it through without being forever changed. And I needed to allow myself to be transformed in that crucible if I was to have any possibility of trying to understand it. There is no stadium seating in combat trauma therapy.

I prepared for this trial the best I knew how. I immersed myself in their worlds. I read incessantly. I watched countless combat documentaries and films. I studied all I could about the Vietnam experience and the turbulence of the American era both inside of and surrounding the war. I learned about the equipment they carried in the field, their tactics, and became fluent in their slang and cultural idioms. I eventually made my own pilgrimage to visit the country of Vietnam, its battlegrounds, and its people.

But most of all, I listened. I listened to the warrior tell their story with my entire being and let them initiate me into their torment.

This initiation happened gradually. So much so that I still, after all these years, can hardly detect its silent presence. But the transformation began with the very first veteran and has not stopped since.

I asked my veterans to lower their guard and become vulnerable. I had to do the same. I opened myself to hearing agonizing accounts I could not unhear and seeing horrifying images in my mind's eye that I could not unsee, all of which I will forever carry. I questioned basic assumptions around which I constructed my world view and challenged my faith in my own invisible "givens." And I had to become honest with myself when a veteran's testimony challenged and deconstructed lies in which I still believed.

As I grew in clinical experience, the descent into my ordeal only deepened. It was not enough to empirically study my worldview—I had to shine that penetrating flashlight inside the deepest corners of myself.

I grappled with who I assumed I was and asked those same exposing questions about the nature of my humanity and that surrounding me. I rejected the myth that only others were capable of the violence we visit upon our fellow beings. I could no longer avert my eyes while glimpsing the beast and human darkness that lies within us all. I addressed the buried guilt that I never served my country in war, and thus was spared their suffering. I eventually accepted that my destiny was different, but my service no less crucial.

I started to dig deep and began to change. I found the courage to become initiated into their worlds, governed by the laws of dark wisdom—the knowledge that one can only claim by journeying through the perpetual, starless night of the underworld, encountering their leviathan, and living to tell of it. And I embraced my own shadow, capacity for ugliness and brutality, and destructive instincts. As I did so, I found humility and no longer felt hampered by judgment.

Once I allowed this transformation to begin, I became more capable of hearing my veterans fully. I developed the fortitude, resilience, and acceptance to welcome their moral anguish and despair. I let them wrestle with parts of themselves they wish never existed without the need for immediate rescue. I watched them struggle and writhe in pain. I embraced their burdens of killing and the taint it leaves behind without rationalization. I shed the human compulsion to rescue others from their suffering. But mostly, I simply bore witness to it all.

I learned that I was more than a healer; I was also serving this community of veterans through development of my own archetypal warrior identity and my initiation into their sacred brotherhood. Only then could I create the trust, safety, and emotional space these men required to look their demons in the eye.

Ultimately, I came to see myself in these warriors. As my transformative process unfolded, I didn't see this book naturally emerge from it. I can't say precisely when the revelation came to me, but eventually it did, and I was humbled by its simplicity—follow your inspiration.

They tell me their stories so that they might heal and, in so doing, touch and inspire my heart like no one else does. That's why I want to write about them. That's why I want to tell their stories. However, what brought me to the place I could share them didn't start when I became a psychologist. It has been a lifelong journey.

⌒

I was born in November of 1968 at the height of the war in Vietnam. As a war baby, I have been attached to this conflict since I was a young boy. I just didn't appreciate it until much later in my life, nor did I see the trail of successive connections that brought me to these veterans.

When I was in preschool in the early 1970s, my father opted to do his mandatory two-year military service in the Air Force. He was given the rank of Major, and our first duty station took us from center city Philadelphia to Grissom Air Force Base in Peru, Indiana. Though I had no awareness of the war at the time, we lived on base next door to a family whose service member was a POW interned at the infamous Hỏa Lò prison, better known to Americans as the "Hanoi Hilton." I played with his younger sons while we were stationed there.

Many years later, I felt compelled to know the identity of this American hero whom I'd never met. I interviewed both of my parents several times, searched for many years, and came to many dead ends. They could remember little of him and could only provide a few clues. Frustrated, I would periodically stop looking only to have the need to find him reawakened over and over.

The completion of my search had to wait nearly twenty years. I recently returned from my own journey to Vietnam in 2016 and visited Hỏa Lò searching for clues of his identity. Our travel group, expecting a basic tour of the prison, was stunned to learn upon our arrival that we were granted an unheard-of, high-profile meeting with Colonel Duyệt, the former commandant during the "American War." I asked him about their higher-ranking prisoners in an effort to narrow the field of names of my officer and former neighbor. Though my visit to that place was haunting and unforgettable, I left empty-handed.

My return from Vietnam reinvigorated my search. Soon thereafter, through the tiniest scrap of information in an archived, small-town Indiana newspaper, I finally discovered his identity. I tracked his latest known, but already dated, address through another obscure Tucson newspaper article. It was a long shot as he would have been in his mid-eighties, but I sent him a letter anyway, explaining my search and the meaning of our "connection" to me.

One day, my office phone rang, and the caller introduced himself as Ron Byrne. It took several moments of mentally scrolling through my patient roster without a successful match before it hit me. Colonel Ronald Byrne (retired) was calling to tell me he was in receipt of my letter and was happy to connect.

I was incredulous my hero was on the other end of the line. I called him that night and this previously unknown stranger told me his story. He told me how he was shot down over North Vietnam on a bombing mission, the details of his capture, and how he was held in captivity for over seven years.

He came home to Grissom AFB for repatriation in the initial phase of Operation Homecoming in early 1973. My mother was standing next to his wife, Joanne, as he stepped onto American soil. This F-110 fighter/bomber pilot, who served our country, endured years of inhuman imprisonment, and who had never met his youngest child, was finally home.

A week after our conversation, I received a personal note and one of Ron's P.O.W. bracelets with his capture date. Worn during the war by Americans back home as a show of support, the bracelets, upon his repatriation, arrived en masse at his home from all over the country. Upon receipt, he fashioned them into a long chain adorning his living room. The one he gifted me is displayed proudly in my VA office. My long search ended with a deeply satisfying sense of completion and a story of war I will never forget.

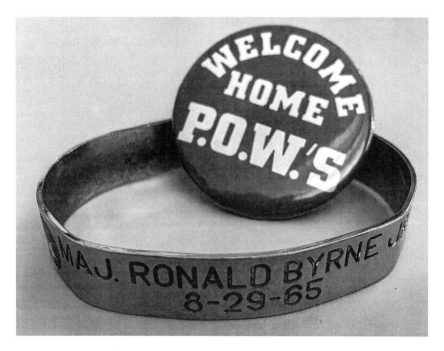

Col. Ronald Byrne's (R) gifted POW bracelet with 1973 Operation Homecoming pin.

I use this experience to counsel my veterans searching for the unknown fates of their comrades in arms, be it in life or death. I tell them this: If you feel you need to search and to know what became of someone important, don't give up. Ever.

Reflecting upon my childhood, I continued to pursue my fascination with military history in general, and of the Vietnam War in particular. My attachment to the war expressed itself through my artwork, its gravitational pull on my interests, and the connections with others that serendipitously crossed my path.

A high school physical education and football coach of mine, Bob Norris, served in Vietnam as a combat medic with 3/22nd, 25th Infantry. He was stationed in Cù Chi, a place I myself visited forty-seven years after his tour. He was severely wounded when his base was attacked by 122mm rockets, and the first barrage directly hit his position. Had he not bent over to pick up an object he just dropped, he likely would not have survived to later cross my path. The rocket exploded just behind him in the barracks and killed half of his unit. It left the survivors riddled with shrapnel wounds. Because he bent over, his vitals were spared while his back, legs, and posterior were filled with the fragments of that rocket.

Coach Norris' athletic shorts revealed his stout legs, one of them appearing as if imbedded with coarse black pepper. One day, my curiosity got the best of me. We stood together in the high school weight room as he picked out the latest piece of that rocket that worked its way to the surface, and he told me the details of how it got there. I will never forget that moment. I will never forget his story.

Almost thirty-three years later, I tracked him down and we reunited for lunch. I wanted him to know he made a difference in my life and that his story, and his combat service in Vietnam, mattered. It mattered to me. Because it did, I dedicated my life to helping his brothers in arms. And that mattered to him.

Other signposts presented themselves along the way on my journey. As a sophomore in high school, I took a summer job at a trap and skeet club. Several of my friends worked there together and we were put under the tutelage of a maintenance man. Though in his early forties, he appeared worn and older than his years.

His name was Clyde, and he was a kind, quiet man who didn't seem to mind our incessant questions and adolescent antics. More visibly, Clyde bore a homemade tattoo on his forearm. In rustic blue ink, it simply read

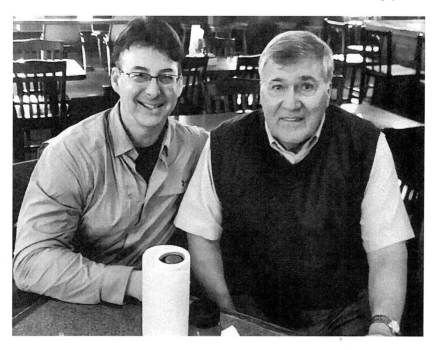

Reunion lunch of the author and Coach Robert Norris, former Vietnam combat medic with 25th Infantry, RVN.

"Vietnam '67–'68." He never said a word about the war, but I found it hard not to repeatedly look at that inscription and wonder what story lay behind that simple declaration. There was also something mysterious about him; he struck me as a man with silent pain hidden behind those gray, tired eyes. But he never betrayed even a hint about what caused it.

Clyde seemed content to have our friendship, no matter our ages. We became rather close and were invited to his trailer for dinner and fishing on the Missouri River. We brought our .22 rifles for some plinking. I didn't know then, but do now, why he flinched when the first volley of rounds knocked the soup cans off the riverbank. After that summer, we parted ways and that was the last time I ever saw him.

I never knew his last name and regretted not having it as I had no way of finding him when it later mattered to me. Had I to do it over again, I would have wanted to hear about his experience in Vietnam. I would have wanted him to know that his service and his story mattered. That someone wanted to know and wanted to listen. However, I just couldn't bring myself to start that conversation. His story, like those of so many other young men sent to Vietnam, will likely never be told. Clyde unknowingly taught me an important lesson—if you care, ask.

After college, I pursued my dream to become a psychologist. I still had no idea where that path would lead. After completing my graduate coursework, I came back home to the St. Louis Veterans Affairs Medical Center for my internship. I discovered something there that felt deeply right.

At the VA, I became involved with Vietnam PTSD groups and experienced the power of men telling their stories in a safe community of other combat veterans. It was my first glimpse into this sacred brotherhood. They spoke of things they would never tell another soul and, in so doing, released their secrets. It was there I learned the maxim "pain shared is pain divided." I witnessed something raw, honest, and magical. The groups helped men communalize the bruise of war on their souls and find the acceptance among one another that they couldn't grant themselves or find in the company of others in their lives. In taking the risk to tell their stories, their narratives became subject to the input of others who knew of combat, and they were able to feel what wasn't safe to feel, or dare express, so many years earlier. This initiated a working through process, and it was helping veterans heal.

I knew then that I wanted to become a part of facilitating this process and help as many of our war-injured as I could. The method was important, but it was the deep relationships, intimacy and sense of connection doing the heavy lifting. Group therapy offered the perfect medium, and it made sense; warriors across all cultures have metabolized the toxins of war and sought healing and resolution in community circles since antiquity.

In retrospect, I arrived precisely where I was supposed to be with the men I was ordained to be with. Their stories inspired me to travel to Vietnam in 2016 with Dr. Edward Tick and his partner Kate Dahlstedt who, for decades, ran healing and reconciliation journeys for war veterans. I felt drawn to see the country and its people firsthand. I needed to look their former enemy in the eye, see the jungle, walk the land my veterans had so many decades earlier, and create a Vietnam in my head that reached beyond the war.

This journey connected my history to the present. I went to Củ Chi where Bob Norris, my high school coach, was wounded. I visited the Hanoi Hilton and met with Colonel Duyệt, the commandant who held my neighbor, Colonel Ronald Byrne, for over seven years in brutal captivity. I met and talked with many of our former enemies. I brought back an honest, firsthand account of the Vietnamese people to my veterans who eagerly awaited my report. For some of my patients, my trip to Vietnam reinvigorated their nightmares as their minds conjured my being killed over there as had so many of their friends five decades earlier. To their relief and my own, I returned home unscathed from this profoundly life-changing pilgrimage.

The author at Vietnam Memorial Wall in Washington, D.C., 2022.

I have learned so much and grown immeasurably from my work with these men. They privilege me with their trust and not just with their hearts, but with their lives. They frequently ask how I could possibly listen to all of their problems and stories. The ones who know me well have stopped asking. They now know the answer.

The truth is, that after all these years, I never tire of their stories, the wisdom they offer, and of the relationships they entrust to me. I feel honored and grateful they granted permission to share the stories of their odyssey and personal transformation with you. I am also pleased to share my own. My hope is that you, too, will take the risk to open yourself to a combat veteran's experience, learn what they have to teach you, and to discover the rewards of this journey.

~

Most of us have never been in combat. We have seen the war movies depicting tortured warriors who returned from Vietnam broken by their experiences. That is not what I found in my work with these vets; most were not broken, but they did have genuine trauma. Instead, I discovered men struggling to impose order on the chaos of their memories and emotions. They sought peace and meaning. Our task in therapy became recrafting a life based not on avoidance of their pain, but an integration of it. This book is organized to bring you through the ordeal of trauma from the Vietnam war and the process of healing those wounds.

Today, it has become commonplace for civilians to speak of carrying trauma. Indeed, over the course of a lifetime, half of us in this country experience an event of sufficient gravity to produce traumatic injury and PTSD. If you've survived trauma, reading about these men and how they worked through their pain might help you along your own journey of healing. To start, you might even find that you can relate to our first veteran, who turned eighteen just days before landing in Saigon. After years of avoiding the war and being scared to ask for help again, he thought he would try just once more.

He had nothing left to lose.

I

The Descent

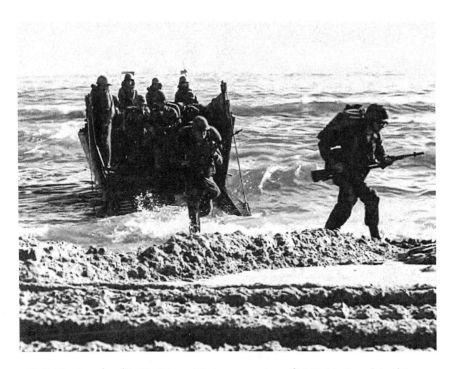

U.S. Marines land in Da Nang, Vietnam, spring of 1965. National Archives.

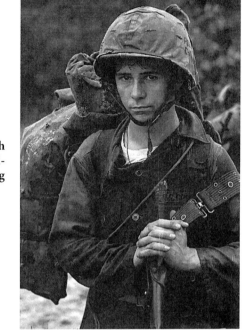

Marine Private waits on beach during first American troop landing in Da Nang, Vietnam, spring of 1965. National Archives.

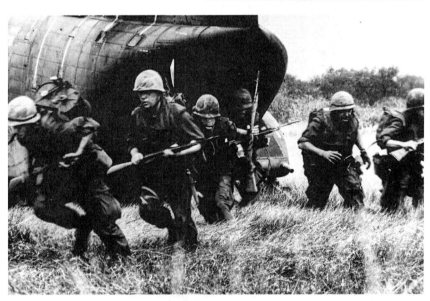

U.S. Marines rush into combat from CH-46A helicopter assault against Vietcong, spring of 1966. National Archives K-31449. Photograph by Photographer's Mate, 1st Class Jean C. Cote.

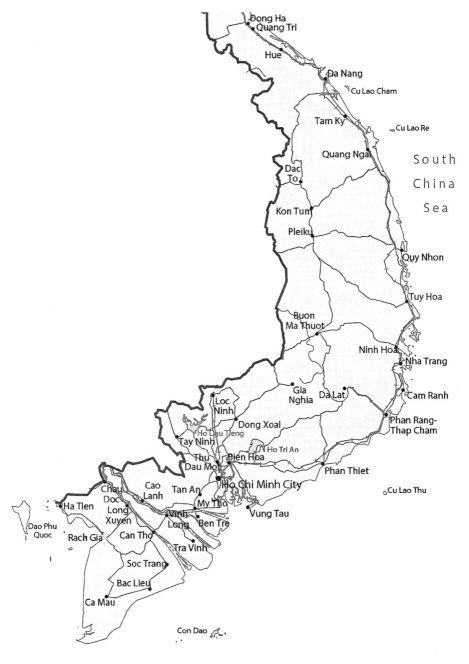

Map of Vietnam. Wikimedia Commons.

1

You're the First

Our eyes locked. This was the moment of truth.

I coached myself not to break my gaze. He was intensely scanning trying to determine if he could trust me.

The silent pause lasted fifteen seconds or less but it felt like an hour as his dark, piercing eyes X-rayed my soul.

My typical consultation interview assumed a natural structure through years of repetition. I didn't know it yet, but he had already crumpled up that outline and laid it invisibly upon my desk. When we got to the tough questions, he refused to give me the information I asked for regarding his trauma experiences in Vietnam. In fact, he announced he wasn't going "there." If he was going to talk to me, it wasn't going to be an interview.

Not this time.

That consultation lasted two hours. Strand by strand, his narrative advanced, cautiously testing for safety every step of the way just as he learned walking point in the jungle. I led, then followed, and

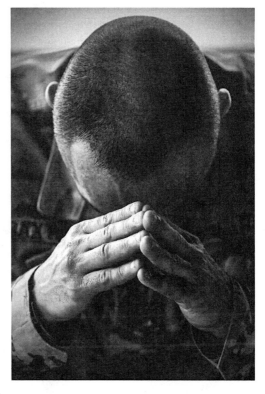

Public domain, RDNE Stock Project.

29

eventually walked alongside him. The winding path was so long and consuming, I almost missed it when we finally arrived.

Before us stood his towering emotional Mount Everest and the awful events in 1968 that built it. Then, in its haunted shadows, his walls, like those of Jericho, disintegrated in front of my eyes. Decades of impacted pain flooded the room, engulfing us both.

After the torrent, we sat, looking at one another, stunned, raw and depleted.

"Is this the first time you've ever talked about this?"

He nodded.

"Cried about this?"

He nodded.

This man had never gone there. Ever.

We sat in unrushed silence. His eyes whispered a blend of tired dignity and gratitude. We reached his underworld, found the lair of his pain, and came through the other side of his ordeal intact. Transformed. And together.

He was now agreeing to treatment after a bad experience with a psychiatrist in the 1990s kept him away from help for almost twenty years. When he entered my office, he didn't let on that this was the last chance he was willing to take. During our meeting, I learned he first came here for help all those years ago hounded by his haunted conscious until he couldn't tolerate it anymore. He capitulated only after he considered his only other alternative.

That day, he had parked his rusting pickup overlooking the river. Tears blurred his view as he toggled between the sweeping vista of the morning fog hovering just over the brown, lumbering flow of the Mississippi, and the blued .45 Colt on the passenger seat. All he could think to tell himself was that it was too pretty a place for a man like him to die in.

Only the sudden bellow of a coal barge's airhorn broke his spell. It was then he turned and saw it through the haze. Perched high upon the river's banks were foggy outlines of the eastern-most buildings of the Jefferson Barracks VA Medical Center. He glanced back at his passenger seat, staring another few moments before more tears came. The 1911 went back in its worn holster and disappeared into the glove box. With a turn of the key, the tired Ford sputtered back to life. He had nothing left to lose.

He sat fidgeting in the clinic waiting room, fighting the gnawing tension lost somewhere between shame and fear. He had never asked for help before, and every second that loudly ticked by on the clock above his head mocked him for seeking it. Just as he stood to leave, a scrub-suited nurse with a stethoscope draped over her freckled neck appeared to escort him behind the locked door. She gestured him into the tiny exam room. The odor of aging vinyl and isopropyl alcohol met him at the door.

"The doctor will be with you shortly." He winced. It felt as careless as it sounded.

He flinched when the metal door latch loudly sealed him into the tiny space. The walls jumped in a few inches when the quiet resumed. He hated small spaces.

Twenty agonizing minutes later, he sprang to his feet as the door suddenly flung open, revealing another expressionless figure in white.

"Have a seat, sir" was all she could muster.

After a cursory introduction, the psychiatrist bombarded him with a hurried series of questions. He tried to answer but was cut off before he completed his sentence. He figured the next question was coming. That's all these shrinks really wanted to know about so they could cover their ass, he thought to himself. He finally lowered his head as he told her about his morning by the river. And about the pistol.

She briefly raised her eyebrows, and then began scribbling on her pad. The pregnant silence that followed compelled his foot to start bouncing again to bleed off the mounting tension in his leg. Then, the cavalier questions resumed. He absorbed one frigid query after the next, until he couldn't.

He broke eye contact, and slammed his fist down.

She had little idea how close she came that day. If she'd known what almost happened, she'd likely been too scared to move.

She jumped at the impact. She pursed her lips, shamed him with her stare and, before excusing herself, pressed the red button hidden under the desk drawer. Moments later, security entered the room and briefed him on her incomplete findings. He was being admitted for a ninety-six-hour "hold" hospitalization, per doctor's orders. He hardly saw the affidavit waved in front of his face. He caught himself watching the hands of each of the officers to plan what might need to happen to get out of the room. In the next moment, he understood—he didn't have a choice.

He clenched his fists in resignation. Never again, he vowed.

But never turned out to be too long.

So, what did he see today for the first time? Whatever it was kept that rage pinned behind the part of him who just couldn't do it anymore.

His penetrating eyes remained, but this time, felt different. Behind them, trust peered out.

I sat, eyes opened to greet it, and humbled to have gained such rare entry. This man, who had carried his pain around longer than I'd been alive, chose me.

He extended a long handshake and something approaching the start of a cautious grin.

He would try once again.

2

War Calendar

"Don't you fuck me!"

He stood in the doorway of my office with eyes that were all business, while his demanding tone barely concealed the pleading beneath it. His gray sweatshirt bore a picture of the three-man bronze statue at the Vietnam Veterans Memorial Wall in D.C., framed in red lettering proclaiming the bitter truth of his sacrifice.

"All Gave Some, Some Gave All."

Ron had to change providers he would see for his trauma therapy. Though our old-school psychiatrist preferred psychotherapy to medications, his caseload was bursting at the seams. I was the new psychologist on the trauma team, and Ron didn't like being forced to take a risk on an FNG. This impasse would be the first of many tests.

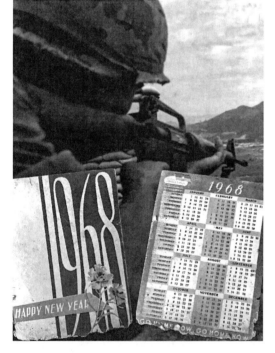

National Archives, photograph by SP5 Dennis D. Connell. Leaflet photograph by the author.

Ron struggled with his combat tour in Vietnam his entire adult life. When he returned home after the war, his stern

32

Slovak mother took one look at him, with tears in her eyes, and painfully asked, "What happened to my Ronald?"

He felt lost after his discharge but tried to follow the road map America handed him. He got a job and started a family. But it wasn't working.

Their home was in chaos. After years of living on his emotional roller coaster, his wife and kids nicknamed him "Dr. Doom." Every year as summer would transition to fall, Ron relived the worst months of his combat tour in lockstep with the calendar. As winter approached, the anguish seeped out of him in alternating fits of rage and bouts of depression. This wave crested just as the end of January arrived, retracing the period of the Tet Offensive of 1968.

While he had many horrific experiences in Vietnam, "the Tet" was the worst. He tried it all. Work. Alcohol. Drugs. When the haze lifted, the memories were there patiently awaiting his return.

They came in disjointed bits and pieces. Some were too vivid while others fused into muted, jumbled fragments. Yet others were recorded from the dissociated perspective of looking over his own shoulder while in the heat of combat, his mind having forced a degree of separation from himself so he could do what had to be done. Over the years, his war coalesced into a horrifying, disorganized mosaic. But the memories always followed the arc of the calendar.

At first, he only hinted at some of what he survived over there. Revisiting it was like staring into the sun too long before its blinding glare forced him to avert his eyes. He would retreat into avoidance and we waited to find another opening when and where he could tolerate it.

When he needed respite, there were other sides of the war he needed to explore—the counterweights of all that had gone wrong. And there were many. If one were to ask him, he might admit pride in his dedication to anything that mattered. Vietnam was no exception. In spite of his traumas, he was no less proud of the soldier he became there. He earned an ARCOM and Bronze Star, both with "V" devices, or valorous action. He saved lives while greatly risking his own. After distinguishing himself in the field, he ascended to driving the jeeps of high-ranking officers and eventually, a general for the 101st Airborne Division. They didn't pick just anyone for those jobs.

However, there was much he wasn't proud of, and that's where we eventually had to venture; we had to go where it hurt. Initially, he doubted he could handle going back to those dark, blurry wounds. And he wasn't yet sure I was worthy of going back there with him.

As we explored the calendar of his combat tour together, our relationship unfolded in a series of slow advances, steep climbs, and perilous plunges. His untamed anger often threatened to derail our journey through his underworld, and old destructive urges easily locked on to people he blamed for his unhappiness.

One day in therapy, he discussed a recent fight with his son-in-law. It got ugly. Had it not been for his grandson's presence to break the grip of his rage, he confessed he might have killed him. In the following session, he broke through to a bitter realization.

"I realized that I don't hate Billy," he reluctantly admitted. "I hate myself."

We dug through several layers before we got to the deeper truth—a truth that men are conditioned from birth to deny. Sessions later, he was ready to say the sacrilege out loud.

"I hate myself because while I was in Vietnam, I was scared. Soldiers aren't supposed to be scared, but I was anyway."

And he had plenty to be scared about.

Ron arrived in Vietnam in late June of 1967 as a replacement with the already seasoned 1st Infantry. It was there he met the beast—those innate, brutal urges that were slumbering inside of him, but were on savage display in the hardened combat veterans surrounding him. They adapted to the unspeakable violence by becoming hunters. They stalked their prey with abandon and adorned their uniforms with macabre trophies. Though Ron didn't know it yet, the violence would consume him as well.

Early in our therapy relationship, he brought a photograph into his session. Ron wanted to show me the eighteen-year-old who landed in Vietnam in the summer of 1967. But it went deeper than that. The oxidizing image depicted the teen soldier, dressed in new jungle utilities wading through waist-high grass behind a bound figure in black pajamas. He proudly escorted his first captured VC prisoner at rifle point to base camp. This moment of achievement, like many in Vietnam, was fleeting and soon interrupted by the bestial nature of this war.

After handing his captive to S2, he learned the prisoners would be transported to battalion for interrogation. Ron watched from afar as their security police escorts loaded three captured enemies into the idling helicopter. They ascended to 1000 feet before slowing to a menacing hover over the tree line just outside the wire. Ron's eyes widened as the soldier he risked his life to apprehend tumbled out of the door like a tiny broken manikin before disappearing into the thick jungle canopy.

That picture told me the story he needed to tell that day. It was his first fleeting triumph during the war, and then the tale of boyish innocence slipping away from him—no, torn from him.

The calendar turned the page into September. It was the month he took his first life. What he could recall of it wore on him, but the blank space that followed bothered him more. He narrated what he could remember before the mental recording suddenly ended.

He was on a squad-size recon patrol near an enemy ville. He saw movement through the dense tree foliage and instinctively shouldered his rifle. The curvature of human form filled his aperture and without conscious command, his finger pulled the trigger.

His heart pounded as the slight-figured youth fell to the earth with a sickening thud. The memory sequence cut off just after the screaming woman he presumed to have been the child's mother, started running straight at him.

For years, Ron saw nothing beyond that opaque crease, which was fine with him. But the unsettling mix of dread and relief that he could see no further refused to leave. He assumed the killing was triggered by the jumpiness of his untested nerves. Such accidents with new guys were common. After the rest of the patrol responded to the rifle shot, Ron stood anxiously waiting for a seasoned verdict as they assembled around the body. Only one grunt cared enough to muster a word.

"Xin Loi, Charlie!" he chuckled before taking out his zippo and lighting his next cigarette.

Ron guessed as to what happened after he shot the kid but didn't want to open the door to what he did or why he did it.

"I think I killed her, but I can't be sure. I don't remember."

No matter the reason, he knew one thing for sure—he didn't volunteer for Vietnam to fight women and children.

It took us a long time to get there. Other events in his tour unfolded before us and took priority for him. At least that was what his shame wanted to believe. But as we entered his fifty-second September after his tour in Vietnam, he couldn't wait any longer. Together, we revisited his first kill.

Ron settled into his chair and tightened his grip on the arms as if to brace himself for the journey. He then closed his eyes and went back to that searing hot day in September of 1967. Like most of his other memories, he watched the scene from over his shoulder, a yard removed from the restless soldier who scanned the ominous foliage surrounding the ville.

Ron talked through the sequence aloud, as if he were walking every jungle-booted step again. He approached the woman's screams of the sudden but familiar ending.

"Keep watching her…," I coached.

Her path unfurled before him.

"Wait…," he paused aloud. He played back the footage in slow motion, but he wasn't sure if it was real, or simply what he wished were true. His jaw muscles perceptibly shifted under his shortly cropped gray beard—he had found something important.

"Behind her ... the kid ... he dropped a rifle when he fell out of the tree."

Like a key finding its mated lock tumblers, something silently, but solidly, clicked. I could see it. I could see him feel it.

I fought the impatience of my curiosity and headed off the question that nearly escaped from me. I took a slow breath and studied his expressions to find the natural rhythm of what was unfolding within him.

"She is screaming at me in Vietnamese. Now she is running at me, and ... she is raising her arm. She has something in her hand. It's ... it's...."

Having found my own attunement, there was no need to ask anything before its time ... because there was no more time. There was only an old warrior facing his dread to find the truth in a story demanding completion.

"It's a grenade ... a chi-com grenade."

The sequence accelerated into the cadence of real time. She rapidly closed their distance. Ron felt his shock give way to primordial instincts before hearing the report of his M16. The shot rang out in his mind as he watched her crumple to the ground, the unarmed grenade tumbling to a halt in the reddened earth.

After exhuming his conscious, he discovered an ending he could better live with. Some clarity helped, but a residue of anguish he couldn't scrub off remained. While it was him or them, the unvarnished truth was that this was his first deadly encounter with the enemy, and it was not what he pictured it would be.

The calendar continued to turn.

Since Vietnam, Ron hated the holidays. We soon came to understand why. The date of one of his citations for valorous action offered the clue he needed to understand why he struggled as Thanksgiving approached. It was the ammo dump explosion, and a day that despite his heroic actions, left the scar of unshakable dread and fear.

As the green treetops gave way to primary hues and the midwestern heat gradually surrendered, he could feel it coming. Raised Catholic, Ron knew of Hell, but never encountered it. That changed in late November of 1967.

With the fire wildly spreading among the ammo bunkers, tens of thousands of crated rounds continued to cook off, firing aimlessly at no one and everyone. Ron raced towards the burning armored half-track, its occupants rendered helpless by heat and suffocating clouds of boiling, inky smoke.

One at a time, he grabbed the disoriented, smoldering occupants, and guided them through the gauntlet to safety, before returning to the inferno. The random death of ordnance succumbing to the flames threatened every step. He repeated the perilous route until the wall of flame closed his path. Through the rippling mirage and shifting shrouds of smoke, he saw no movement in the charred chassis.

There was nothing further he could do, but it was the searing question that his bronze star couldn't answer. It was the same question vexing all who survived the impossible when others didn't.

Could I have done more?

The answers hid in places foreign to the warrior ideal. It required confronting the ideas military training sought to destroy—messages so unassailable that they didn't register as beliefs, but of universal law: they were taught they were omnipotent and invincible. They were convinced before they were deployed that they could do anything. While that message prepared them well for hell, it did nothing to rescue them from surviving it. Little did he know the ammo dump wouldn't be his only trip into its fires.

Ron's night watch post sat upon a sandbagged bunker overlooking the sprawling air base at Biên Hòa. For weeks, military intelligence uncovered signs that an attack on this massive base was imminent. Long-range reconnaissance patrols from the 51st Infantry intercepted two enemy recon units probing the area just north of the base. Something was brewing, but both sides negotiated a cease-fire in honor of the Tet Holiday.

Air base security remained on 100 percent alert yet again, but that heightened alarm wore on the exhausted troops in III Corps; each warning followed by another uneventful night on the perimeter lured the weary troops into complacency. While word of some isolated attacks in II Corps filtered through the RTOs working in headquarters, so far in their sector, all was quiet.

Ron strained to keep watch on the perimeter, the dancing shadows toying with his senses and emotions. Nighttime in Vietnam had a way of fucking with a man.

His duty partner lay propped against the sandbag wall, not even pretending to care what might be out there. He showed up for his watch stoned and it wasn't long before the rhythmic ballad of crickets and cicadas lured him into a careless slumber. Ron found his irritation distracting as he struggled to keep his heavy eyelids from obscuring his view of the concertina wire.

He called in with his last radio check to deliver yet another negative sit-rep. He could hear the distant crackle of fireworks as the nearby city of Biên Hòa welcomed the Lunar New Year. It was the night of January 31, 1968.

The faint "whoosh" of the 122mm rockets gave way to a deafening explosion of the jet fuel depot that shook the earth. An immense mushroom cloud of boiling flame lit the darkness.

Ron recounted the unbelievable sight in session. "I literally thought the world was ending…," he said in a half-whisper with dilated pupils offering a haunted window into the opening salvos of the Tet Offensive.

His night watch partner jolted into wakefulness and gripped the sandbags to steady the world of terror into which he had just been thrust. Wailing sirens sparked a chaotic scurry of half-dressed soldiers pouring out of doorways trying to orient themselves in the fire-lit night. Men looked to someone, anyone from whom to take orders. The explosions gave way to the disjointed symphony of overlapping, automatic weapons fire. Panicked red tracer rounds searched for targets. The attack they were told might be coming for weeks, and grown exhausted from expecting, was here.

That mushroom cloud disintegrated the higher ranks who were supposed to know what to do but, in the opening moments of the brazen attack, didn't. Now, they were just men—shouting, hyperventilating, and stricken with the same frailties as the soldiers beneath them.

Ron ran towards the sounds of fighting coming from the besieged side of the air base. The USAF security forces were manning that bunker line. By the time the officers coordinated a response, the enemy overran the perimeter and took up positions in those bunkers. The intruders turned their fury towards the interior of the base to confront the mounting counterattack. The previous defenders in those vanquished bunkers now littered the floors.

Ron joined the firing line of American troops forming in a ditch in front of him. He could feel the unforgiving, perforated steel surface of the Marston mat digging into his kneecap as he knelt and took aim at the infiltrated bunkers.

While changing magazines, Ron recognized the balding, un-helmeted American next to him. He was one of the few men he remembered as kind and likeable. He talked to him several times on base and even knew him on a first-name basis. His name was Fred.

In the next moment, that balding head exploded in a pressurized pink spray of blood and brain matter. Before Ron could fathom what happened, he instinctively wiped his eyes of the sticky film so he could continue to fire. He didn't have time to do otherwise.

The popping cacophony of automatic fire filled the air, blotting out everything but the screaming. The screaming of orders, of the wounded, and of the madness of battle.

And then, almost as quickly as it started, the gunfire from the bunkers began to falter, and then stopped.

"Cease fire! Cease fire!!"

The order travelled up and down the line as deafened men stopped shooting. Acrid smoke hung in the air. All that could be heard was the metallic sounds of rifle actions cycling, the changing of magazines, and the slamming of bolts on freshly charged weapons. In the lull, Ron turned to check on Fred.

There was perfectly round, bloodless hole in the middle of his forehead. The back of his head was gone. The full weight of the horror didn't hit him until later when he discovered that his uniform was covered in pieces of one of the only men in Vietnam he knew on a first-name basis.

The American line cautiously advanced.

As they neared the first bunkers, a black-pajamaed survivor with a bamboo conical hat and an AK-47 in hand fled towards the outer wire. Ron reflexively shouldered his weapon and fired a burst into the enemy's back. The impact spun the figure into the concertina as the bamboo hat slid off to release a long, flowing mane of black hair.

The American line got low, paused and then slowly made their way towards the eerie silence of the pock-marked bunkers. Ron apprehensively approached his kill. He looked down at her fixed, empty gaze before reaching the other men now clearing out the bunkers.

Ron was absorbed into the hastily assembled Task Force Ware that assisted in the fight to retake the American embassy and, eventually all of Saigon. After several days of heavy fighting, on February 4 the task force arrived at the Chinese district town of Cholon (Chợ Lớn) the west bank of the Saigon River, where the VC remained stubbornly entrenched. After evacuating most residents and declaring the entire area a free fire zone, the town, constructed almost entirely of wood, was bombed and napalmed into charred skeletons and ash. Ron's unit sifted through the smoldering ruins, going house to house, pulling out the bodies.

I looked at his face as the haunting spell of his story lingered in the room. Ron's dilated pupils constricted as the adrenaline began to subside. Though his harrowing experiences didn't end after the American's ultimate victories during the Tet Offensive, it was that time period during the first half of his tour that consumed him. We would have to revisit that awful place many times throughout his therapy.

As he processed his memories, he began to heal. He likened our work to peeling an onion, because the metaphor of many layers surrounding a deep core seemed fitting. As he worked through each painful layer, the fumes of the war stung his eyes.

I couldn't say exactly when it happened, but one day, we found ourselves at the very deepest core of himself. And I couldn't say how long after that Ron stopped hating himself. Then, slowly, he began learning to like himself.

One day he walked into my office, smiling. He pointed at his face and said, "Hey Doc, look…. I think I finally learned how to live with one."

⌒

"Don't you fuck me!"

As he stood in my office doorway, I sat evaluating his stern warning not to betray his trust. I saw his angry, but vulnerable eyes. They were asking the most important question he could ask of me. He wanted to know, after all who had betrayed and lied to him, if I was trustworthy.

He stood in the threshold of my office door, neither in nor out. The three-man statue and its red-lettered testimony telling the story behind his despair. Though Ron survived the war, he gave it his all, sacrificed parts of himself to do so, and paid a dear price ever since. He was now asking what I was willing to put on the line in order to help him.

He cautiously accepted my invitation to close the door and have a seat.

Now I talked. He listened.

I offered him this: I knew trust was earned and that he could observe me—watch to see if my words and actions matched, study me for truth-telling, and see if he could count on me.

He seemed satisfied with that pledge. But our contract wasn't yet complete. I needed a commitment from him too.

"So, tell me, if we were successful in our work in therapy, what would be different in your life? How would we know we accomplished our mission together?"

He paused and thought for a moment. He leaned forward over the edge of my desk to make sure I heard what he wanted. His eyes and voice stated it with the piercing sincerity that I came to cherish among my combat veteran patients.

"I've been depressed and angry ever since I came home from that place. I must have survived for something worthwhile. I need to believe that. So here is what I want—I want to die with a smile on my face."

I paused to consider his proposal before leaning to join him over my desk.

"How about instead of dying with a smile on your face, you try living with one?"

He thought for a moment. His pursed lips melted into a smirk, and his eyes softened just a bit.

"Ok, you've got a deal."

3

The Grunt with One Name

"Where do you feel it in your body?"

Jackson clutched his chest and winced, locating the epicenter of his decades-old hurt. He coughed nervously in a futile effort to clear the feeling that was bubbling up from his core.

For months, we worked on the spotty narrative of his primary trauma in Vietnam. The overall storyline fell into place, but he had left out a big piece. Jackson's eyes shown with hurt and confusion.

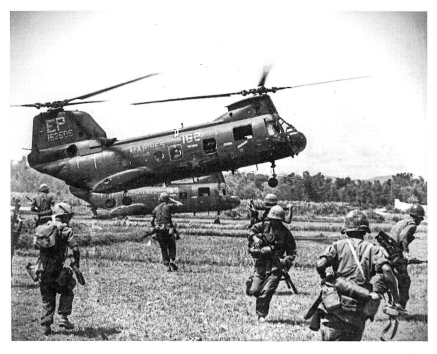

Marine CH-46 Sea Knight extraction, Wikimedia Commons, photograph by R.C. Hathaway.

"I am not sure why I keep thinking of this guy who I barely knew."

His name was Bryant.

Because Marines went by last names in the field, it was the only name he could remember. Bryant was a replacement who just rotated in the day before the mission that changed Jackson's life forever. Untested and green, it was never easy for replacements.

Most of the grunts didn't want to know your name until a man proved it was worth knowing. Much of the time, they died before that happened, only cementing the code further into place.

Unlike the other old hands in the platoon, Jackson was not going to push Bryant away to keep a safe distance. Jackson recognized that his seven months of surviving in Vietnam with the 1/7th Marine Infantry was worth something and that it might keep this new guy alive. Then, he reasoned, one day Bryant might return the favor.

Survival logic aside, he and Bryant hit it off from the start. They were both Midwesterners rendering them virtually kin in this strange world so far from home. In session, Jackson reflected upon their brief time together to fill in the gaps.

"I knew him for less than twenty-four hours. He was from Illinois. I remember that. We were in base camp, and we could relax a little. We couldn't know that the very next day, we would both have the worst day of our lives."

But for now, they were in the rear. They talked for hours, went to the PX for cigarettes and candy and, due to their mounting comfort, even briefly left their weapons in the deuce-and-a-half as they walked to indulge in some cherished luxuries. The relationship deepened quickly without regard to the mere hours of togetherness.

The buzz made its way through the ranks. Orders were coming down, but they had nothing solid yet. Soldiers facing death soon learned just how valuable even some brief time out of the field could be. Jackson cracked a smile as he reflected on those precious hours. There weren't many times during the war he could smile about.

"That day, life wasn't so bad considering we were in I Corps in Vietnam."

Early the next morning, they were lined up on the company street readying to board the idling helicopters. They were told only what they needed to know—nothing more. They were going on a rescue-recovery mission and would seek the downed pilots that, according to military intelligence, had survived the crash.

They were going to rescue Americans. That was all they needed to know.

The enemy was near. How near didn't matter.

They were Marines.

Semper Fidelis.

Jackson and Bryant lay face down behind a sunbaked rice paddy dike. Between the downed pilots and the Marines lay the enemy. Command ordered an infantry assault on a tree line across an expanse of open ground—a frontal attack. After leaving this lone dike, there would be nowhere to hide. Jackson's fireteam was on the far-right flank of the assault line.

In session, Jackson reflected on those last moments of safety.

"Was this excitement, fear ... what was I feeling? I wasn't sure. It was so confusing. All I knew was that I was going to do my job and hopefully finally see and kill my enemy." The feelings fought their way up his throat forcing another fit of coughing before venturing back to the paddy dike.

When it was time, word traveled up and down the lines. Then, they jumped up and started running.

At first, all he saw was the menacing jungle edge, bouncing with every stride. Jackson heard nothing but his labored breath and the sound of equipment-laden men charging the unsettling stillness of the tree line in front of them. Out of the corner of Jackson's right eye, he saw him. Bryant was running too.

The edge of the jungle suddenly awakened with flickering flashes, and less than a second later, erupted in a violent roar. The fire came from everywhere, the world exploding around him. The enemy were dug in, surrounding the enveloped Marines on three sides. Invisible angry hornets pierced the air around Jackson's head as he ran straight towards the darkened trees, the flashes betraying his hidden foe. Jackson focused on the pulsing flicker directly in front of him and accelerated his charge.

Suddenly, within scores of yards from his objective, he fell.

He paused the battle, and further reflected:

"At first, I wasn't sure why I stopped running. I tried to force myself to my feet but was unable to stand—my left leg wouldn't work. For decades, I blamed myself for not reaching that tree line, fearing that I had not done my job, had let down my fellow Marines, and had not lived up to my expectations of myself."

The deafening chatter of battle suspended time as he searched his body for the reason. He discovered a bullet pierced his thigh and exited his buttock. The blood soaked his utility pant leg while he dispassionately watched it spread, curious as to why there was no pain. An enemy machine gun burst yanked him back into the war.

Jackson looked up. He saw Bryant running hard towards the tree line, just as he had told him to do.

Then he saw him fall.

The battle intensified as the assault teams closed in on the edge of the jungle. Under their cover, a corpsman sprinted towards Jackson. Bullets nipped the air as he applied a compression dressing and, with the assistance of another Marine, battle-carried him to a waiting CH-46 Sea Knight helicopter in the distance.

They traversed the gauntlet to the awaiting bird as the dead and wounded were evacuated to the landing zone. The rotor wash whipped the dust and dead vegetation into a tornado of debris. At the rear loading ramp, Jackson gave away his rifle to another Marine who was still in the fight, but in the chaos of battle, lost his weapon. He watched as the others who were capable hurriedly threw the row of lifeless bodies on the helicopter.

Screaming over the roar of the accelerating engine, the crew chief herded his passengers aboard. The wounded did as they were told. They scrambled up the ramp and piled into a tangle of bleeding humanity on the floor.

"We didn't have time to treat the dead with the reverence they deserved—we were still under fire—a hot extraction. We had to get out of there."

The twin rotors of the Sea Knight whirled in a frenzied pitch to generate the lift needed to escape. Bullets pierced the chopper as they cleared the ground making two distinct sounds as they entered and then exited the thin metal skin.

"Thunk ... thunk ... thunk ... thunk!"

The metal hull crisscrossed with haunting beams of sunlight tracing the trajectory of relentless ground fire. There was no mistaking it now; Jackson felt the fear coursing through his body. Joining the cacophony, the deafening roar of the door gunner's M60 opened up to cover their escape.

The aircraft climbed and banked to the left, gaining distance from the battlefield. As the sound of the fight faded, Jackson's adrenaline-fueled mind slowed just enough to register the jolting sensation of what was underneath him.

He couldn't bring himself to look down. But he didn't have to.

He was lying on his fallen brothers—men who shielded him and the other wounded from ground fire as their bodies absorbed rounds coming up through the floor.

Jackson couldn't resist any longer. He owed it to the Marines that had saved his life even in death. He forced his eyes beneath him and looked at two of the lifeless faces turned towards him.

One of them was Bryant.

~

Epilogue: Bryant's identity remained a mystery for years after the veteran opened this traumatic memory—after all, he had barely known him before he was killed. However, Jackson needed to know his friend's name so he could properly lay him to rest in his mind. Using the only available scraps of information and with the assistance of the veteran's spouse, we found the man previously known only as "Bryant."

His name was Michael Steven Bryant. He was twenty years old and hailed from Des Plaines, Illinois. Bryant was a private first class, replacement 0331 (machine gunner) of 1/7th Marines, 1st Marine Division. He joined Jackson's outfit just before 1/7 deployed for Operation Desoto on January 27, 1968. This operation was a relief mission to rescue the crew of a downed aircraft in Quảng Tín, Đức Phổ District. The 5th Marine regiment began the rescue and Jackson's company was flown in to assist in the assault. While they moved down the hill towards the wreckage, they received heavy small arms fire from the north, south and west. Taking heavy casualties, the Marines pulled back. During Operation Desoto, four Marines were KIA and nineteen WIA. The four dead Marines were Marvin Bennett, Sidney Fleming, Nicholas Navarro, and Michael Bryant. Michael Bryant is buried in the Towne of Maine Cemetery in Park Ridge, Illinois, and is honored on the Vietnam Veterans Memorial Wall, Panel 14E, Line 85.

4

Blue Eyes

All of these years later, he still doesn't understand why he wound up on a small dusty combat engineer compound near LZ English in Vietnam.

Sure, Allen was in the Army, but his MOS was supposed to place him on a NIKE anti-aircraft missile base. Though he was no expert on the strategic deployment of U.S. missile assets around the world, he was unaware of any such bases in South Vietnam.

When he arrived in country and handed over his orders, it wasn't long before he was on a deuce-and-a-half traveling towards Bồng Sơn where he would serve in support of the 1st Cavalry and later, the 173rd Airborne Divisions.

The Army never trained Allen as a combat engineer, but he soon discovered that his primary job was keeping Highway 1 "open." This highway was the main travel artery through the heart of South Vietnam. It was also a primary target for local VC forces hoping to disrupt the constant flow of troops and war material.

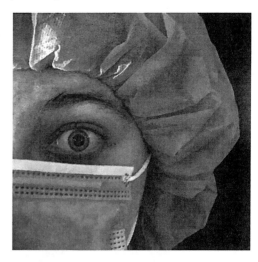

Mining the road was the enemy's strategy of choice. The counter strategy was to go out every morning with mine detectors to clear the road of mines. Allen's detail would eventually meet another squad of engineers as each worked from their end of the highway until they met somewhere in the middle. At that point, they could declare the road "open."

Author's photograph.

46

Open, however, was often fleeting. This by no means meant the road was safe. The VC had elevated their favorite tactic, the combined arms ambush, into an art form and cost American forces dearly. The surprise attack began with either a pressure-activated mine or command-detonated explosive followed by small arms. Once they disabled the lead vehicle, the road was no longer "open" and anyone unfortunate enough to be caught in the kill zone was in trouble.

That's how Allen lost Michael, his best friend. They were pinned under a vehicle trying to seek shelter from the fusillade of bullets slicing through the kill zone. Michael wasn't supposed to panic, jump up to leave cover, and take off running. But that is exactly what he did, and within only a few steps, he was struck by a bullet in the neck and died right there on the side of Highway 1. The road had been "open" a minute before they killed Michael. Allen watched helplessly as bullets kicked up the dusty earth.

Michael was, according to Allen, just a good person. He was also married and had someone he would now never come home to. Allen shook his head reflecting on the senseless loss. "He didn't have any place in Vietnam—he shouldn't have been there."

The pain behind his voice suggested that he was not the only one who shouldn't have wound up in Vietnam. But the day Michael was killed was only one of the many things Allen experienced that he wished he hadn't.

Pulling guard in Vietnam was sometimes more a matter of protocol than practicality. On moonless nights, it was often so dark that a person could not see their hand in front of their face. Allen questioned the utility of guarding a perimeter he could not see against a possible ground attack he would never know was coming until it was too late. However, this did nothing to disrupt the necessity of guarding the wire.

On just such an opaque, inky night, Allen found himself on watch. He was straining to stay awake and relieved to have successfully finished his shift without giving in to the sleep impatiently waiting for him. However, his replacement never bothered to show up.

He figured the NCO whose responsibility was to monitor the changing of the guard would eventually make his rounds of the perimeter, discover the break in protocol, and promptly correct the matter. It soon became clear that no one was fulfilling that responsibility either.

Allen sat with his dilemma in the smothering blackness—no one was coming. In Vietnam, figuring out what and who you could count on was a daily struggle.

He remembered his drill instructor making an example of the pitiful recruit next to him for making that mistake once during basic training: A soldier is never supposed to leave their post until properly relieved of duty. But Allen's exhaustion eventually won out, and he set about finding his replacement himself.

He slowly maneuvered towards the direction of his bunker with his hands out in front blindly searching for clues of his location. He eventually found the familiar contours of stacked sandbags which signaled the entrance of the bunker in which he and the other engineers lived.

Allen walked his hands along the dank, gritty wall of the entrance. He felt the shift in the bags of the interior corner in the passage as it turned to the left. His hands guided him through the familiar mental map of the reinforced bunker. Inside was his duty replacement and some desperately needed sleep.

Behind the concertina wire, the network of claymore mines and machine gun bunkers, the men who lived on that thinly defended base learned that, in Vietnam, one could neither be too safe nor too careful. In the darkness, Allen felt the slight flex of a thin wire tighten across his palm.

In an instant, the stillness of the night exploded. The startling combination of the assault on his senses and the pain shooting up his arm jolted him from exhaustion into the sudden mobilization of everything.

He vaguely recalled the alarm of others and the scurry of activity after the blast, but his cone of attention quickly focused on the sensate awareness of the searing pain of his injuries.

"I remember looking at my hand—it was smoking."

He was airlifted to the 85th Evac Field Hospital in Qui Nhơn , about eighty-two klicks SE of Bồng Sơn.

The triage area was crowded with the wounded, many more severely than Allen. He watched from his stretcher as nurses scurried among litters of men in agony as the surgeons attempted to repair their broken bodies.

Allen faded in and out of consciousness, caught in the swirling haze of pain and anesthetic. His memory of the hospital had more holes than cohesive pictures. But one image would endure for decades after the war.

Standing at the foot of his litter, he made out the angelic silhouette of a scrub-suited nurse. As she leaned in close and extended some human comfort to assuage his pain, the limited features of her face left uncovered by the surgical cap and mask came into sharper focus. And that's when he saw them.

"They were the most striking blue eyes I had ever seen. They were almost purple. But it wasn't just the color. There was a kindness in them. That was the first and last time I'd seen kindness in anyone's eyes in Vietnam."

When he awoke in recovery, he searched for those eyes among the regular shift changes of hospital personnel. He never found them again.

Allen's memory of the days following his surgery was spotty. He recalled that there was a POW camp adjacent to the hospital and that the entire facility was evacuated during his convalescence due to the imminent threat of an enemy attack. Other details he couldn't forget. He could still see and hear the horrific injuries of the others and the sounds of suffering that mercilessly wafted through the wards at night.

Those disjointed pieces simply bled into the suspended nightmare of the war that picked up just where it left off upon returning to the field. After his hospital discharge, Allen rejoined his unit in Bồng Sơn. He noted a strange, but palatable silence; no one—not an officer or fellow enlisted man—said a word to him about what had happened that night. There were no answers about who had set the booby trap in the bunker's entrance or any mention of ordered changes in how men on that base dealt with the constant fear of being killed.

Nothing.

So, Allen just went on about the business of trying to survive another day until his time was up. He would go on to confront death on many occasions during his remaining time there and have many memories carved into his mind that he wished he could forget. Just about the only memory of Vietnam he didn't care to discard was that of the compassionate, anonymous blue eyes in Qui Nhơn.

⁓

Allen knew something was wrong upon coming home from the war but struggled for years to cope—alone.

His wife was unable to tolerate anything about Vietnam. She lost a cherished cousin over there, and her pain shut the door on that war and everything related to it—including her husband.

Allen was no shrink, but he put together that her chronic anger and biting criticism of him was likely an unconscious rage and below that, grief; he survived while her cousin had not. And because of the deep well of guilt and shame Allen carried from the war, he believed that he deserved whatever she aimed at him. This Faustian bargain kept them together but locked his despair firmly in place.

Allen went from doctor to doctor trying to keep painful memories of the war at bay. He followed every prescription promising relief, but none of them could heal the bruise on his soul. He eventually found his way into the VA for treatment and one day, while we were in a therapy session, he described an encounter he had several years earlier.

Allen began his story by recounting his wife asking him to mail an important package in advance of the approaching holiday season. For him, what sounded like a routine errand was anything but.

Allen struggled with intense anxiety when in public. He lost his basic trust in other human beings a long time ago. As a result, the ever-active radar for the unexpected kept his nerves on edge to the point where even a simple outing could become intolerable.

He adapted the best he could. He learned to position himself with his back to a wall and located the exits within moments of entering a new structure. He couldn't stand the sound of footsteps coming up behind him. He simply stopped and pretended to adjust something as he let the stranger pass him by.

The deeper truth was that Allen was never sure if that person was in pursuit with intentions to harm him. While it sounded illogical, if not ridiculous, when he said it out loud, he learned not to leave such matters to chance a long time ago.

The dots weren't hard to connect—when your own men, who you must trust with your life, come close to killing you, it damages the inherent faith in others. This shakes the very foundation that holds mankind together—the invisible compact of social trust and assumed good intentions of other people. Since Vietnam, Allen no longer enjoyed such luxuries.

As he sat in his truck at the Post Office, he could feel the anxiety escalating. The parking lot brimmed with impatient customers in the waning days of the holiday rush. Wedged between his fear and the argument with his wife for a failed effort, he cautiously approached the door to his local branch.

Upon entering, Allen's eyes darted in a futile attempt to track the flurry of activity. But it was too much: Too many people. Too much movement. Too much noise. The overstimulation engulfed him. His pounding heart joined the sweat beading on his forehead. He knew immediately.

He had to get out. Quickly.

As his truck's door closed solidly beside him, a slowly fanning wave of relief spread through his body. It didn't last long.

The unsent package sat pitilessly in his lap. He conjured her face, etched with disappointment as the surge of adrenaline worked its way through his system. Sweat breached his oversaturated brows and ran down the gullies of his cheek. The sickening spiral of fear clawed its way back.

He fumbled for the container of pills. He washed one down with the lukewarm coffee in his truck's console, its familiar bitterness offering promise. He leaned back, closed his eyes, and waited....

In minutes, Allen felt the elusive peace wash over him. At the hospital, they taught him to slow and deepen his breathing to augment the welcomed calm. The spinning gears in his mind gradually began to catch again, and, within a few minutes, he was able to redirect himself back to his dilemma: he could not go back in there, but he also could not go home with that package.

He was surprised it came to him that quickly, but it was a good solution.

The Post Office in a neighboring town was far smaller and out of the way, but that was the point. As he pulled out onto the two-lane road, he had already inserted a plausible breakfast stop into the storyline he was rehearsing.

He pulled into the tiny lot in front of the modest federal building, A wry smile spread to welcome his good fortune. There were only four cars in the lot and one customer was already heading for the classic Chevrolet Camaro convertible on his right. Being a car guy, he found himself sizing up the vintage based on its butternut yellow original paint before he realized he was habitually finding something, anything to avoid going in.

He sat weighing his odds for a few moments as another customer left the building, but Allen didn't want to press his luck. He took a deep final breath, tucked the package tightly under his arm, and cautiously walked through the front door.

In fractions of a second, Allen sized up the small rectangular room. The analysis came back clean just as quickly; there were no threats present. With his back now exposed, he instinctively perked his ears listening for anyone entering the building behind him. No one was there.

In front of him, an elderly man on a walker waited behind the young mother with her impatient toddler who was at the counter quickly pouring over her options for Christmas stamps. Allen felt the strangeness of the novel room merge with a growing sense of hope that could return home with success. He couldn't remember the last time he felt that way.

The old man offered a holiday greeting as he placed his giftwrapped box on the counter, and the postal clerk began the procedure of getting the package to its destination. Allen watched as she worked. Her methodical movements absorbed his attention until her voice broke his spell.

"Thank you and Happy Holidays…. Next…," came the flatly toned pleasantry.

Allen obediently approached the counter. Though he rarely looked directly at another person when speaking to them, Allen could not help but to be transfixed as he got the first close look at her face. Her mouth betrayed no hint whatsoever of an emotional state, and though one was not required to work at the Post Office, it stood oddly in contrast to the nearly omnipresent holiday cheer.

He didn't realize how long he had been standing in front of her, as he was distracted by the growing stir in his gut.

"What can I do for you today?" she asked with a hollow intonation.

The question jolted Allen back into the present moment. However, parts of him were trailing behind as they worked the incomplete puzzle. He assembled her features into a familiar gestalt, but it didn't fit anything he had on file. He heard a voice, sounding like a distant recording of himself, say that he needed to mail a package. He then watched his arms, as if they belonged to someone else, mechanically rise to offer it to her.

As the clerk processed the package, she briefly returned Allen's gaze. He reflexively averted his eyes to break the awkward intimacy.

Allen was disoriented by his straddle of the past and present. The desperate search through his memory gave way to a kaleidoscope of pictures, the appearance of which came with a tinge of nausea. Scraps of memories appeared, were disregarded, and then quickly reassembled. He felt his stomach drop and his mouth go dry when the final piece fell into place.

He had a match.

It suddenly became clear why he couldn't place her facial features—they had never been available to begin with.

Neither was the graying hair, nor the deeply etched lines that revealed a woman who had long struggled, in parallel to Allen, with her own hidden anguish.

Her blue eyes were almost purple—the decades had not changed them one bit.

Allen reeled against the sheer odds. Never in his thirty-six years of living in the area had he set foot in this tiny Post Office in the rural town adjacent to his. Though the likelihood seemed impossible, he couldn't leave without knowing for sure.

Doubt and anxiety crept in as he weighed this uncharacteristic risk. His thoughts insisted on retreat. Somehow, he felt his feet root to the tile floor. He swallowed hard to find his voice.

"Excuse me, this will sound strange, but I think I might have known you a long time ago … did you serve in Vietnam?"

The woman pivoted to put the package in the bin behind her. She paused too long before gradually turning and staring directly into his terrified, eager eyes.

The kindness he remembered that once belonged to those deeply blued irises had long-since vanished, along with many other ebullient qualities the young and naïve Army nurse brought with her upon arriving in the Republic of Vietnam in 1966. She went there to serve her country and help others. Like so many Americans who did the same, she got more than she bargained for.

A century passed for Allen since his question, but it had been but a mere instant.

Her haunted eyes finally locked with his.

Under her breath, in monotone and without a shred of emotion, she nearly whispered,

"Qui Nhơn … 85th evac…."

And then, without another word, she dropped those blue eyes, placed the "closed" sign on her counter, slowly turned and walked away.

5

Welded Wings

It was more of a shrine than a home office. Though I never saw it in person, while we sat in session, he described his sacred space with pride. Pictures, memorabilia, and various sentimental treasures testified to his history of passions and spoke with authority to the most influential experience of his life.

While Marco was proud of his eight years of military service and two combat tours in Vietnam, the collection's focal point celebrated the warrior he became over there, and the enduring gift of his two best friends that shared that journey with him.

Marco served his first tour in Vietnam with the 44th Rangers in a

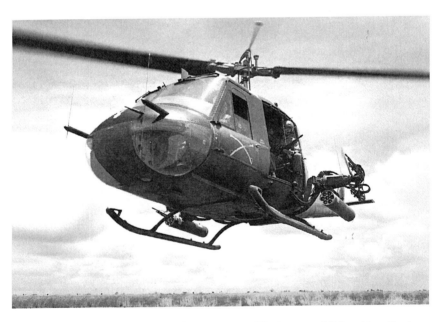

UH-1B "Huey" Iroquois, United States Army Heritage and Education Center.

recon unit operating out of Bạc Liêu in 1968. However, he wanted to fly helicopters in combat and soon found himself at Ft. Walters for rotary wing flight school. Flight class 69–34/69–30 was learning to fly on a TH-55 trainer. Those who succeeded would go on for additional training on the warbirds they would eventually fly into battle.

In flight school, Marco met many other aspiring pilots, one of whom was Gary Frasher—a name that later intersected with his life in ways he could have never imagined. But it was there at Ft. Walters that Marco also met the two men whose friendships he would cherish for the rest of his life.

He knew it from the moment he met them—Skip and Merlin were special. From the start, there was an undeniable chemistry between them. The trust among the trio set in quickly and cemented them into inseparability.

It was everything Marco valued; there was authentic connection, camaraderie, a flowing ease of togetherness, and no bullshit. When they weren't learning how to fly, they were sharing time together, having fun, and fortifying their bonds.

But it was something deeper that attracted Marco to these men. He earned his Combat Infantry Badge and had been to war, leaving the precious innocence he saw in his two friends somewhere in the jungle. When they went out for the night after a hard day of training, Marco quietly marveled at their glow and the ease with which they both embraced the simple joy of living.

Merlin was the socialite. Lead by his boyish smile, by the time he left an engagement, there was not a person remaining in the room who couldn't count him as a friend. The addition of their wives made them into a cohesive sextet. While Marco was with Linda, Skip and Merlin were both with "Kathys." The six of them grew closer by the day. They were making plans for the future—a future together.

Flight school was demanding and while some in their class were not destined to be pilots, the three friends excelled. Demonstrating those skills in solo flight was the final stage of training at Ft. Walters. The trio celebrated their graduation in the customary way; one by one, after they successfully soloed, the friends were tossed into the pool at the local Holiday Inn. From there, it was off to Ft. Rucker.

These men were being prepared for a different kind of war; a guerrilla war where they fought an elusive enemy and inhospitable jungle terrain. Both conspired to thwart the movement of a modern mechanized military and offered the enemy the dense cover to launch sudden hit and run attacks before melting back into the landscape.

The military planners answered with a strategy pivoting around the concept of "air mobility"; men would be flown in and out of battle in helicopters. The UH-1H Bell "Huey," and the men who flew them, became the strategic centerpiece in Southeast Asia and America's first helicopter war.

Unlike Marco, Skip and Merlin had not seen war. They hadn't encountered their enemy or hunted for him in the bush. They hadn't been shot at or felt the nausea wash over them after their first kill. They hadn't confronted the complex feelings that arose in a man fighting for his life and doing what was necessary to keep it. And they couldn't appreciate what was awakened in a man who was going back.

When their flight class gathered to watch documentary footage of the nature of combat in Vietnam, Marco stepped out of the room. The other men responded to the carefully selected images and the reflexive thrill of going to war. The rush of flying choppers into battle surged through their veins. They projected themselves onto the screen and imagined victory.

That was not what Marco saw. Old feelings surfaced out of the depths of his gut. The jungle on the screen suddenly came alive and enveloped him with the sounds of bullets cracking as they flew over his head, the yelling of men in battle, and the acrid odor of cordite hanging in the humid tropical air.

Marco tried to remember what it felt like before he went over the first time—the intoxicating spell invading the imaginations of young men heading to war; men who had yet to fight in one. He didn't have the heart to take that innocence away from them. He knew where they were all heading would claim it soon enough.

The trio completed their training and earned their coveted wings. Marco, Skip, and Merlin were now rotary wing pilots and heading for combat duty in Vietnam.

In late 1969, their orders came with a mix of excitement and sadness. They bid farewell to their ladies and readied for deployment. They'd be back, they assured. And their wives took comfort in what they saw in their husbands. They wore their brimming pride and confidence like their newly awarded pilot's wings. The indomitable strength of the weld between the three men only added to their aura of invincibility.

Though they all knew where they were going, only Marco knew what that really meant. He didn't come out of the jungle feeling invincible. But he couldn't bring himself to think too long about the possibility of being killed in Vietnam, and so he allowed his deeper fears to be swept away by his friends' naïveté. To Marco's recollection, the subject never came up among the three of them—not once.

These young warriors were in the prime of their lives. They were trained to pilot the most technologically advanced weapons system of their era. They felt bulletproof and the Army flight instructors did all they could to build that illusion.

And they had the wind at their backs; this training seamlessly poured into the rushing torrent of their youthful masculinity. The three of them were striving as young men do; striving for adventure, striving to be tested, and striving to conquer the ultimate archetypal rite of passage a man could undertake: they were going to war.

Marco sat in session reflecting on this image. The mental snapshot of these bonded friends, full of life and courage, were embarking on the same path as had so many men before them—the mythical hero's journey. The underworld awaited them.

There, they would undergo the silent initiation that would change them forever.

Marco paused for a moment to savor that image of them together. He stared into the darkness of their adventure as he continued to tell the story of this trio's journey into the abyss.

Skip landed in Vietnam just ahead of Marco and Merlin. Upon arriving in country, the great demand for helicopter pilots split the three friends as they headed to different units. Marco was sent to the 7th/1st Air Cavalry out of Vĩnh Long. He and Skip would fly the Bell AH-1 "Cobra" gunship, America's first production attack helicopter.

It was late 1969. Though Marco missed his friends, the frenetic pace of the war and the intensity of its demands first distracted him, then consumed him.

When the war wasn't demanding his attention, Marco dreamed of the life that awaited the three of them. He caught himself remembering the good times, the laughs, and the promise of a future filled with more of the same. But the hard duty made the days and spaces in between melt into one another. He nearly missed the calendar turning into the next decade.

It wasn't long after that he got the news.

Shortly after arriving in Vietnam, Skip was flying his first combat mission on January 27, 1970. He was with a highly experienced instructor pilot on a nighttime "phantom" counter-interdiction mission in the U Minh Forest near Cà Mau.

Their objective was to strike targets along the canals the enemy used for the transport of war materials under the cover of darkness. Skip's Cobra descended through the low cloud ceiling for a gun run to engage their third target when they collided with the tall trees of the triple canopy forest. The aircraft exploded on impact, killing Warrant Officer Wes Carrol and 1st Lieutenant Theodore "Skip" Leighton.

His death devastated Marco. But there was no time to grieve—the war wouldn't permit it. He couldn't forget, nor could he dwell. He continued his job and to the extent that some of those feelings found their way into the course of his duty, the enemy paid a price.

Paid for taking his best friend. Paid for the pain. And paid for changing Marco's life forever. Everyone knew how it worked. It was the way of the war: don't get sad—get even.

A month-and-a-half later, Marco received a letter. It was from Merlin. He was assigned to the "Little Bears," A Co. 25th Aviation Battalion, 25th Infantry. While he was stationed only 167 klicks to the north from Vĩnh Long, it felt a million miles away.

Marco felt the wave of sadness wash over him again as he read the letter. Merlin was reaching out to share his grief with the only remaining man on the planet who would feel like he did. Though the connection was reassuring, Marco knew it would never be the same after that; their triangular bond cracked.

But at least he still had Merlin.

In session, Marco could hardly stand to talk about it, and yet he couldn't avoid it for long either. Skip's picture was prominently placed in his office shrine, and the grief was never far. Sometimes it surfaced when we discussed Marco's history of troubled relationships. Other times, it appeared as one acquaintance after the next fell short of Marco's standards for friendship.

The bar was high, and one prospect after the next failed to meet them. While not unrealistic, the standards were simply unfair—no one could ever fill the boots of his fallen friend.

His unrelenting grief dwelled like a ghost unable to leave the haunted edifice holding his earthly pain. In session, when a seemingly unrelated topic brushed against that emotional nerve, the impacted mourning would erupt out of nowhere.

Only it wasn't from nowhere. It lived deep in his heart—it kept score and an eye on the date. The ache came every time the calendar turned a new year. While others celebrated the birth of a new year and its promise, Marco was reminded that several short weeks later, he lost one of the best friends he ever had. After January came reprieve.

That is, until May came.

In 1970, Mother's Day fell on May 8. For the rest of her life, that holiday would forever become the day that another Gold Star mother would mourn the loss of her son.

It was also the day Marco would henceforth associate with the death of his second-best friend, Merlin.

On May 8, 1970, the final weld broke. Marco was now alone.

Though it was forty-five years later, the hurt and loneliness remained. He sat in smothering agony as he told the story of losing his two best friends. Though he fought it, tears flowed into the forest of his gray beard. His eyes sought relief on my busy office wall. Searching for something that might offer a moment of distraction. He abruptly changed the subject, looking for escape. Anything to avoid the hurt.

But it never stayed away for long. The calendar always brought it back.

For fifty years, Marco believed the version of the story that filtered back to him at Vĩnh Long; Merlin was shot down while running an emergency resupply mission. Out of his ship's crew of four, only one survived.

Several years after I first heard this story, Marco received a letter. The author introduced herself as Joan, the younger sister of Merlin's slain co-pilot and aircraft commander, 1st Lieutenant Gary Frasher. She was seven years old at the time her brother died in Vietnam.

Frasher.

Marco froze when he saw the name. He, Skip, Merlin, and Gary had been in flight school together at Ft. Walters. Destiny brought them together once again.

For years, Joan searched for Marco. She attended a military reunion hoping to locate some of her deceased brother's comrades in arms. One veteran she met there provided his address.

He didn't get much personal mail and his curiosity broke the seal on the envelope with no forewarning. Though she was a stranger, and Marco had long ago grown wary of strangers' intentions, he hung on every word while navigating a torrential flood of feelings. Marco could hardly believe what he was reading.

Joan recounted the day her family learned of Gary's death. She watched her mother nearly collapse when a government car pulled in front of their Iowa farmhouse and saw the men in their pressed green uniforms solemnly step out of the vehicle. By the time they left, her mother was never the same.

It hurt to read the letters, but Marco couldn't avoid them. It was a connection—his only living link to his slain friends.

Only, it wasn't. Or, at least, it didn't have to be.

Marco felt himself recoil at the invitation. Joan offered to put him in touch with Merlin's surviving sister. She almost lost him there; the proposal smashed into walls containing his grief. It was just too close.

When Marco reported this offer in session, I could hardly contain myself. I'd seen other veterans make similar connections with surviving family members and, most often, healing followed. I wanted it for him, but it wasn't my call.

He shot down whatever hopeful expression I wore. I took one look at Marco and knew this meeting was never going to happen.

He couldn't imagine enduring such a painful reunification. Marco met Merlin's sister in 1970 while attending his stateside funeral. He scrolled through his memory and pictured the young girl in black seated in the front row as Merlin's mother's trembling hands accepted the triangularly folded flag.

He shook his head attempting to dislodge that intolerable image. He couldn't imagine awakening that agonizing day. Or his enduring grief. No, he would continue his correspondence with Joan, but not a single step closer to his pain.

All of those years, Joan struggled with restless questions of her own. She dug into her brother's past trying to understand why Gary didn't come home to her. During that process, she not only found Merlin's sister, but discovered critical details of the circumstances surrounding their brothers' deaths.

The official story suggested that Merlin's chopper responded to a resupply call to aid an engaged infantry unit fighting on Hill 284 in Tây Ninh province. However, Joan's research found this unit didn't need a resupply and, according to available records, never radioed to request one.

What she discovered didn't make sense, but once she told Marco, he connected the dots. He grimaced at the emerging picture.

"The enemy would do that sometimes," he explained in session. "They would use our radio frequencies and make resupply requests in English. Then they would lay in ambush."

Marco stared at my office wall to steady himself. It was a busy patchwork of art, keepsakes, Native American crafts, and war memorabilia. It was also a perfect mosaic to distract a man from what was happening inside. It brought him too close to that day he lost the last best friend he would ever have. He felt another wave coming and tried to anchor himself to wall.

But it was too late.

For him, it was Sunday, May 8, 1970, once again.

The fraying strands that were about to connect all of these Americans to one another hadn't yet felt the imminent rupture of Merlin's death.

That day, tail number 69–15058 answered the resupply call.

That day, 8,470 miles away in Worthington, Iowa, Joan and the Frasher family were trying to make the best of Mother's Day in the awkward void of Gary's absence. His mother got through it by promising herself that, next year, they would be together again.

That day, in neighboring Nebraska, Merlin's mother mustered a smile as her family wished her Happy Mother's Day. Underneath her pursed lips, she whispered a prayer that this day next year, she would once again feel the radiant warmth of her son's boyish grin.

That day, Mrs. Leighton's faced her first Mother's Day without her Skip. It was the first of too many.

For a 7/1st Cavalry cobra pilot, it was just another day of war. Another day of beating the odds. Another day of taking the fight to the enemy. Another day of staying alive.

That day would change everything for all of them. These Americans, most of whom never met one another, and whose paths would have never crossed, were welded together by love and loss.

Forever.

6

Flower of the Heart

Joseph sensed the end might be near. During the night, he awoke gasping to catch his breath. Soon, despite his exhaustion, he dreaded his awaiting sleep. He wasn't sure he would wake up.

Even at seventy-three, his frame still bore all the markings of a formidable warrior. He had worked as a high school physical education coach and retired after a long fulfilling career. As an avid hunter and woodsman, he searched for a plot in the country where he could spend the rest of his days enjoying his passion for the outdoors. Eight years ago, he and his wife found a little piece of heaven in rural Missouri where he built his home, tended his garden, and spent most of his time in the hardwoods teeming with wild game. It was his Garden of Eden, a domicile of natural beauty, and a home he never wanted to leave.

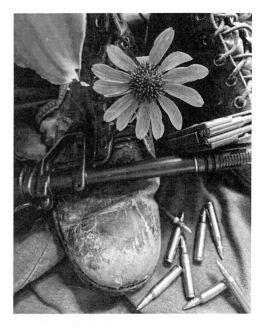

But paradise required maintenance. His body and mind still wanted to work, and there was always much to do. It was his heart that wouldn't let him.

His cardiologist implanted his pacemaker on the left side so Joseph could still fire a rifle, but one thing after the next went wrong. They tried to tame his recalcitrant arrhythmia with several ablations, multiple

Author's photograph.

62

medications, and electrical shocks. The physician was methodically working through an ascending protocol of options, but nothing was working.

The COVID-19 pandemic wasn't helping. Joseph was hospitalized three times to treat his arrhythmia since the coronavirus invaded America. Because he was at high risk, every episode of medical care upped his odds of an invisible final blow. Though he was used to spending much of his time on his property, he was now more isolated than ever. He was struggling to make sense of it all.

Joseph wasn't scared of dying. He lost that fear a long time ago in the jungles of Vietnam. Like many warriors, he resolved his fear of death so he could do what had to be done. That meant hunting his enemy and taking lives—it was his job, and the lives of he and his men depended on it.

These were the facts of war and, for him, the conclusion was simple: when your death came, there was nothing left to do but embrace it.

It was just your time.

The truth was that he was more concerned about *how* he would die. During the war, he saw too many young men perish horribly. Some of those deaths blurred into the fog of war. Others were so vivid, so personal, and so gut-wrenching, he couldn't escape them no matter how hard he tried. This was especially true for Will.

Joseph never got over Will's death. It didn't matter if it was his time. When Will was killed, a part of him vanished forever—it broke his heart. Years later, this fallen brother in arms would come to him in his nightmares, standing in the shower washing the blood off his youthful body, and trying to assure him he was okay and now in a better place.

Joseph wanted to trust that. He believed in God and tried to let his faith salve the loss. He knew it must have been Will's time. But the pain was still there.

In Vietnam, Joseph was the only one in his unit who graduated from Army Ranger school. His skills were in high demand, and he served in elite reconnaissance units with both the 5th Special Forces group and the 4th Infantry Division. As a Sergeant of Fox Force, he wore the burden of leadership with a balance of confidence, good judgment, keen combat instincts, and humility. His men knew it, respected it, and because of it, followed him anywhere.

He needed their devotion. Recon was a high stakes gamble. Their job was to find and eliminate the enemy—they were hunters. They operated in enemy territory for days at a time: stalking, watching, and listening. They traveled light, mastered camouflage, used small unit guerrilla tactics, and melted into the surrounding jungle. If their prey was small and vulnerable enough, they would lay in ambush. Other times, when outnumbered, they observed the enemy, let them pass, and radioed in their positions.

And sometimes they became the hunted. The "men with green faces" were earning a fearsome reputation, and the allied South Vietnamese Army honored each man of Fox force with a cherished red scarf for their exploits on the battlefield. The enemy offered a handsome $10,000 bounty for any American killed wearing one.

Whether one was predator or prey depended upon many factors, but none more so than the element of surprise and correctly judging the size of the opposing force. Like hornets, it was hard to know how many the nest held. But a leader had to get it right or people died.

With a silent hand signal, the recon patrol reflexively squatted in the bush and became one with the jungle edge. Joseph low crawled up to his point man. The whisper was barely audible.

"We've got movement." His point man was motioning down towards the valley below.

Joseph always led from the front. Without a sound, he slithered through the foliage and took a position behind a small shrub. From this high ground, he could see where the jungle gave way to a sprawling, lush valley.

It was then he saw him.

The young North Vietnamese Army soldier was walking straight towards him. His gait was unhurried, his posture casual and unguarded. His pith helmet partially shadowed the upper half of his face from the relentless sun. A soiled khaki uniform hung off his thin frame. Oblivious to the concealed threat lying in wait in front of him, his AK-47 was harmlessly slung upside down over his shoulder.

He was half-stepping in the bush—a dead man walking. It was almost too easy. This was hardly the first unsuspecting enemy that had walked into his kill zone. He silently slid the safety off.

But that was not what caught Joseph's attention.

It was the wildflower that the NVA soldier held up to his nose; its perfume drowning out, just for a minute, the stench of the war. The fanciful smile he wore punctuated his naivete. Joseph calmly followed him through the aperture of his rifle sights.

The battle-hardened tactician weighed in first. Joseph scanned past the approaching NVA. He now saw movement in the valley below. Steadily advancing, khaki uniforms multiplied against the dense emerald foliage.

Emerging out of the brush were a couple of black-pajamaed Viet Cong carrying captured American M16s. That image gave Joseph pause. The anger bubbled up within him as he imagined the fate of the GIs who had once fielded those weapons. The team's advantage continued to dwindle as more khaki uniforms filtered through the tall grass. Joseph felt the odds shifting. They were outnumbered and couldn't risk giving their position away.

But he wasn't going to let them pass unscathed either. They caught the enemy out in the open. There was going to be a fight.

He continued his battlefield calculus. They had the high ground, the element of surprise, and a weapon more deadly than the enemy's superior numbers. They had a radio. Joseph quickly recalculated. The warrior tactician in him smelled victory.

Another side of Joseph surfaced as his eyes fixated on the wildflower in the soldier's hand. He didn't care much for half-steppers—they got people killed. But there was something about that flower.

The soldier's steps slowed, and his image blurred as time screeched to a standstill while Joseph's attention turned inward to wrestle with his decision. To pull the trigger of his CAR15 and kill him, Joseph had to blur this young man into a target. By this time, it had become almost involuntary. Again, the flower came back into crisp focus and the soldier's slow stride gradually accelerated until his cadence slipped back into real time.

No. It didn't seem right for a man to die like that.

Joseph felt the tension of his trigger finger ease. He watched as the NVA followed the crease in the earth to his right and gradually disappeared behind a grassy knoll, utterly unaware of how close he had come.

Joseph took a deep breath, exhaled and gut-checked his decision for a moment. His heart answered. It came back clean.

The sudden crack of rifle reports broke the silence and echoed through the valley. The shots came from the rear of Joseph's observation point. Without any deliberation, he knew exactly what had happened as his brain instantly assembled the situation.

Awaiting Joseph's sit-rep and orders, two of his men on the left flank had spotted the enemy point man as he rounded the far end of the knoll. From their rear position, they wouldn't have seen the awakened nest in the valley below.

Khaki uniforms came from everywhere. The distant muzzle flashes gave a second of silent warning. Then the air filled with the raging cacophony of automatic weapons and the frenzied dance of green and red tracers.

Their surprise now gone, there wasn't much time. Bullets kicked up the earth as Joseph returned fire. His squad filled the firing line to his right and left in the well-orchestrated counterattack. The RTO joined Joseph on the line and quickly presented the handset that would call in the fire support they needed.

It wasn't long. The distant thumping reverberated off the valley's steep walls. It was the sound of salvation for the pinned down team, and the fight raged against the rhythmic background of the inbound gunship.

The Huey's M60 machine guns soon dominated the fight. The crew expertly worked the valley floor, chewing up everything and everyone in their path. The green tracers and distinctive clacking of AK fire gradually dropped, wavered, and then trailed into silence as the gunship made one gun run after another.

The fight was over. The pungent smell of nitrates and haze of gun smoke hung in the humid tropical air. All that could be heard was the bold thumping of the Huey blades above, proclaiming victory.

Joseph and his men looked up and offered a grateful wave as the helicopter made its final pass. The pilot triumphantly dipped a skid to reveal the crew chief in the gun well returning a thumbs-up before it peeled off and headed home.

The chopper's echoes gradually lessened until the valley resumed its stillness and eerie silence. The team began their descent to take stock of their quarry. Khaki uniforms littered the ground as they searched the dead for intelligence and began the routine of counting. Some officer in the rear was waiting for a tally of captured weapons and bodies. And many miles away, several people above him were waiting for the same.

As the team started the macabre task, Joseph looked to his left at the grassy knoll. It was the last place he had seen him. He stared at it for a moment. He just had to know.

Joseph surveyed the heading he imagined the point man would have taken after he disappeared from view. He put in a fresh magazine and pulled back the bolt to ensure he had a round chambered. Then he followed the crease into the valley.

His tuned senses scanned ahead. He silently rolled the heel of his jungle boot into every step, looking for anything out of place. As the ground cover thickened, he saw the fresh path of disturbance through the vegetation. He had come this way.

Joseph glanced up towards his vacated fighting position to triangulate the place the point man would have first reappeared when his team fired upon him. He replayed the time that had passed until he heard the opening shots of the battle. He wiped the stinging sweat out of his eyes before looking up the hill to confirm his final calculation. The enemy soldier would have emerged just about ten meters ahead.

Joseph sharpened his stare and opened his senses. He didn't see or smell any blood. There was no metallic glint of a dropped weapon. He couldn't see a khaki uniform or any movement through the thick underbrush. Then he froze.

His mind raced and he crouched to lower his profile. His ears perked and strained, listening for any sound suggesting he was now the hunted.

The earth was still. He detected nothing. He scanned the surrounding brush again before gingerly approaching the target spot ahead.

Something was out of place. His gut tightened, and then loosened as his body instinctively judged no danger. His adrenaline-fueled muscles released, and his clenched jaw relaxed before breaking into a leery grin.

A smile ... out here. It felt odd, but good at the same time. It was the first he could remember having for far too long. He walked over to the spot, stood straight and stared down as he turned inward, the ground blurring beneath him.

The swirl of feelings confused him. This point man was his enemy, and given the chance, one who would have killed him. Joseph could have easily cut him down, but didn't. And if he was being honest, he wasn't sure why.

He replayed the firefight but the answer wasn't there. And his conscious was clean. Of all the enemy he had killed, he didn't hold any regrets. But this one was different—he didn't *want* to shoot that man.

Why had he traded his rifle for a flower? Joseph let the answers find him.

Perhaps it was his exhausted nerves, scanning the endless trails for threats that were at once nowhere and everywhere. Maybe it was the leaden burden of the killing or of braving the oppressive heat, the relentless elements, and the jungle. Perhaps it was the pit of homesickness in his gut and the image of his girlfriend that wouldn't leave. Perhaps it was the smothering grief of watching his friends dying in agony just feet away. Joseph felt the painful truth in each projection.

Or was it just the moment a soldier took notice of the beauty all around him. Joseph had felt the same temporary intrusion of sanity; there were many times in the Central Highlands he suddenly become aware of the native allure of the jungle, ignoring the madness of warring men. He, too, had made the same mistake of noticing how beautiful the world could be just when he might be leaving it.

The ground under his jungle boots came back into focus. Joseph reached down to pick it up and held the flower to his nose as it shared its fading perfume. Joseph smiled to himself again as he turned to join his team.

It just wasn't his time.

7

Cost of Courage

He couldn't believe it was finally over. He watched his platoon saddling up to head back into the field. This time, he wasn't going with them.

Paul was a short-timer. With only four days left in his twelve-month tour, he was granted permission to stay on the tiny fire base until his orders came in. He didn't think to say goodbye to anyone he fought alongside of before they disappeared once again into the surrounding jungle. He was leaving Vietnam the same way he came—alone.

To celebrate his going home, the young crew chief popped a smoke

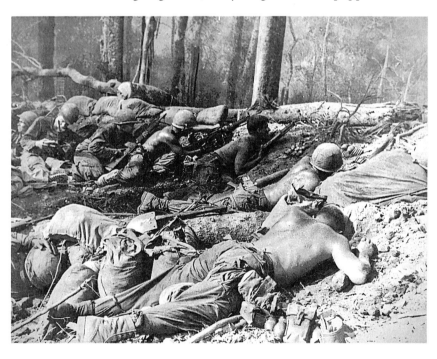

U.S. Army photograph.

68

grenade attached to the skids of the ascending Huey helicopter for his final ride out of the bush. Paul watched numbly as the shrinking soldiers on the ground waved in salute of the red smoke trail signaling that another one of their own had made it out of this place alive.

He wasn't sure what he felt anymore, but he told himself he'd be okay now—he made it. However, like the red clay caking his rotting jungle boots, he didn't realize the war would follow him home.

Fifty years later, Paul's profound emotional isolation came from the impossibility of conveying to another person what being scared to death for a year will do to a man. Or the way the fear still smothered him. He struggled even with other Vietnam combat veterans because most of them wouldn't admit they were *that* scared out there in the bush. Paul didn't have that issue—he couldn't deny it. The fear was still, all these years later, far too real for that.

He lost count of the times he said "no" to social invitations to venture out of his limiting safety zone. He gave up responding to the quizzical or disappointed looks of friends and family who couldn't understand his polite refusals. When his shame became too heavy, he tried to participate once more only to succumb to his fear's grip yet again. They didn't understand that it had nothing to do with his love and devotion to them all.

It was about one thing and one thing only—the fear. It had trailed him out of the jungle, permeated his soul and fundamentally altered his way of being in the world.

It wasn't always this way. As a child, Paul learned to face down his fears. He was taught to stand up for himself and protect those around him. He detested people who used their authority to exploit and abuse others. And he fought when he had to.

But this was different. This was no schoolyard bully. This wasn't a neighborhood ruffian in the alley shadows. It wasn't fear of a single thing, place, or person. It was the lurking terror of being hunted and the constant threat of annihilation. It was everything and everywhere.

Paul was drafted into the Army in 1969. It was also his first real encounter with the use and abuse of institutional power. They trained him to be a soldier but this was no democracy; he would have to do what he was told, go where he was told to go, and fight who he was told to fight. Just like the young men to his right and to his left. And like most of them, he didn't really understand the guerrilla war he was being forced to fight in Vietnam. Paul had no idea how far into hell this obedience would drag him. Nor had he any notion of how terrifying the journey there and back would be.

Upon arriving in country, the war began its assault on him. The stifling heat and humid air carried the indescribably putrid odor of refuse, death, and decay. Random sounds of distant fighting echoed off the rugged and deceptively beautiful landscape. Scattered columns of smoke billowed towards the cumulus clouds hugging the mountain tops. The tropical sun intermittently broke through and mercilessly beat down upon him and the other green replacements.

Wide eyes strained to see what was coming as they were hastily prepared for war. With deadened efficiency, supply clerks issued the new guys their gear and sent Paul to a holding company until receiving his assignment. He didn't know it yet, but he was being sent to the 4th Infantry Division. It was better he didn't know.

The 4th's area of operations was the mountainous Central Highlands. This particularly punishing terrain was blanketed with a dense, triple canopy jungle, honeycombed with caves, tunnels, and a sprawling network of foot trails. There were an infinite number of places for the enemy to hide, and to attack at times and places of their choosing. The land and climate foiled much of the modern American Army so it became an infantryman's war.

In the jungle, men devolved and hunted one another like animals. Paul had never been preyed upon, but his nervous system quickly adapted—a transformation that began upon reaching his unit and didn't stop for the next twelve months.

His company's orders were the same as those who hunted them—find and kill the enemy. His unit's leaders kept the 22nd Infantry Regiment out in the boonies until they accomplished their mission or died trying. Paul's fear only grew as they traversed the ominous jungle foot-trails of the Vietnamese Central Highlands, while being pursued by an enemy that was often hidden until it was too late.

Paul stared at the breadth of these well-worn earthen paths carved through the jungle one footstep at a time. He imagined how many steps it took to erode the earth and beat back the untamed undergrowth. He visualized the generations of Vietnamese men who traveled down these very routes fighting one invader after the next for a thousand years. The descendants of those men now hunted the Americans. Despite punishing losses, they didn't show any signs of giving up as the generals had promised.

Paul noticed the sickening dread the first time his column began to move down these jungle pathways. But he wasn't out there by himself.

An infantry line company was hard to conceal. Soldiers on the move were only as quiet as their noisiest man. And there were too many of those. Some made commotion because they were "half-stepping," their complacency maddening; with their level of experience, they should have known better—half-stepping in the bush was a death wish. Some because they were FNGs and hadn't yet learned how to move through the jungle. Others were simply beyond caring anymore. And some made noise because it was impossible not to.

Their infantry company carried an immense amount of equipment, each with its signature sound broadcasting their position to anyone within earshot. Half-empty canteens, unsecured rifle sling swivels, heavy rucksacks, grenades dangling off nylon web gear, and men frequently losing their footing in the mud and entangling jungle floor all joined the heavily armed chorus.

An infantryman man struggled not only under the weight of his own ponderous load, but also carried his share of the unit's common equipment: mortar rounds, iron base plates, hundred-round 7.62 M60 ammo belts, and M72 LAW rockets. As the mission wore on, every ounce weighed on a man's depleting stamina and will. But that was only part of the risks they took every time they went outside the wire.

Paul also questioned the wisdom of some of his leaders. It didn't make sense to him to move this clamorous column down the well-worn jungle trails in pursuit of the enemy who created them—this was Charlie's backyard.

Paul strained to stay quiet every time leadership decided to use the enemy's own trail system for another operation. Then, they would lock and load, and set out for another patrol, their equipment-laden bodies bumping and scraping as their hunting party made its way through the jungle.

Exhausted, the column reached its objective before the unmistakable sounds of setting up camp resonated throughout the mountainous landscape. The metallic clanging of shelter poles driven in with steel helmets, the sharp echoes of entrenching tools breaking into the rocky earth, the acrid smell of cigarettes and of cooking decades-old C-rations over flaming tabs of C4, all wafted through the forest.

And Paul noticed it all. Every sound, every smell, every unnatural movement, every man he wished was paying attention as much as he, but wasn't. His fate was tethered to those men, and so he learned to pay attention when they weren't.

That is how he first saw the two VC fighters using shadows to stalk the bivouacked Americans. He detected movement. His heart began to pound.

In silence, they moved like panthers through the underbrush before disappearing behind a thick old-growth tree. Paul slowly raised his rifle and waited. In the fork of the tree, he saw the rising curvature of a head. When enough of it appeared in the peep sight of his M16, he squeezed the trigger. The shadow limply folded behind the trunk, while palm fronds snapped back into place covering the escape of the lucky one. The crack of Paul's rifle's report raised the alarm of his now-alerted unit.

It was his first kill and the critical lessons followed. Watch, look, and listen. Never drop your guard and, above all, be ready.

Be ready for anything. Be ready for everything. Always.

It was a lesson his nervous system would never forget. He didn't know it yet, but this vigilance was to become the indelible script for his life. The hunted had now become the hunter. That's how he was going to make it home.

Paul never relished the killing. But it wasn't much of a choice, really. He stayed in the bush his entire tour in an endless search for an elusive and relentless enemy. Better them than me, or so the saying went.

Though the 4th Division unofficially operated across the Cambodian border, leadership finally became frustrated enough to authorize an invasion. In early May of 1970, the 22nd Infantry and many other combat units on the western border of Vietnam, pushed into neutral Cambodia to attack the previously off-limits North Vietnamese sanctuaries. The loud drone of advancing men and material traveled for miles. As they pushed inland, signs of the enemy were everywhere.

While Paul didn't care much for some of his leadership, he did like the twenty-two-year-old junior officer in his outfit. He won the men's admiration because he cared for them and made decisions accordingly. Because of this, he was one of the few officers Paul respected.

On May 7, while searching a fresh bunker complex, they were ambushed. During the ensuing firefight, this vaunted officer and another infantryman were shot. Paul helped carry his lifeless body to the medevac chopper. Word filtered back that his officer died shortly thereafter. The loss hit Paul hard.

They hacked an LZ out of the wilderness, brought in supplies, and built a fire support base around it. Command tapped Norse lore and named it "Valkyrie" after Odin's female guides of slain warriors to Valhalla. It was a good spot. While modest in size and early in construction, the bases' high ground, defensive bunkers and fighting positions offered more cover than the 22nd were used to. Several 105mm and two 155mm howitzers complimented the mortar section at the center of the perimeter adding some welcomed firepower and reach into the surrounding enemy sanctuary.

The 22nd Infantry were in the NVA's backyard but, as was common, the enemy refused to engage. Cloverleaf patrols searched outside the perimeter and intensified their hunt. The men weren't going to get sad about their earlier losses—they were going to get even. Frustration replaced the fading promise of payback as the guerrillas dissolved back into the jungle.

As was typical of the war in Vietnam, a chain of men beginning thousands of miles away were deciding what came next. The North Vietnamese had long taken sanctuary in Cambodia and Laos, knowing the Americans could not politically risk widening the war. When President Nixon finally announced what was true for years—American forces were operating in Cambodia—the anti-war movement exploded. Shortly thereafter, the war-weary executive leadership issued orders to withdrawal just as Americans forces closed in on their primary objectives and were accomplishing the tough job they were sent to do.

Less than a week after Paul's favorite officer was killed, orders came down that they were pulling out of Cambodia and returning to their AO inside Vietnam. In preparation for their relocation to An Khê, command ordered the deconstruction of the camp. Nothing was to be left for the enemy.

Word passed down the ranks—they were pulling out in the morning. The sounds of equipment and hundreds of working hands permeated the surrounding forest.

They struck at about 3:00 a.m. Explosions rocked the earth.

During the initial wave, a combined arms attack rained rockets and mortars inside the perimeter. The deafening blasts were punctuated by automatic weapons fire and the piercing screams of besieged and disoriented soldiers stricken with fear. Parachute flares turned the deep blackness into a haunting magnesium-illuminated scape of terror. A heavy .51 caliber machine gun located on a nearby wooded hill attacked the west side of the base with streaks of glowing green fire.

Americans rushed into their partially dismantled perimeter bunkers, taking cover in its remnants, and shooting at shadows and muzzle flashes. Only the violent exchange of green and red tracers streaking through the darkness separated friend from foe. Command ordered the perimeter defenders to stay in position less they mistakenly shoot one another in the dark. To repulse the attack, artillerymen lowered their tubes and fired devastating beehive rounds directly into the enemy ranks. Shredded men disappeared into their blasts.

Paul's pulse raced as he took his firing position. In the midst of flickering pandemonium, something inside their perimeter didn't fit. His darting eyes caught a crouching silhouette that made his heart skip a beat. The short figure sprung to his feet, running towards the command bunker. They were in the wire.

Paul raised his rifle, sighted the sprinting form, and dropped him with a controlled burst of 5.56mm fire.

Paul stared at the peach glow slowly rising through the trees. He didn't believe he would live to see it again. As dawn broke, the macabre debris told the story.

The smoldering earth outside the wire was strewn with broken pieces of men and blood trails. Orange embers glistened in heaps of rubble and ash. An indescribable odor of smoke and stench of things no longer living hung in the humid air. Dazed survivors silently mulled through the detritus. Miraculously, while many Americans were wounded in the attack, only a single artilleryman was killed.

The Captain was making inspection of the line and the courageous defense of Valkyrie, and the NCOs made their reports. Paul learned that the running man he killed was an enemy sapper. He stopped him before delivering his deadly cargo. The bodies of the sappers, adorned only in loin clothes with charcoal darkened skin, were laid near the chopper pad. The Captain congratulated Paul on taking down this crucial trophy.

"Is there anything I can do for you, soldier?" the Captain offered.

"I could use a R&R, Sir." Paul half-joked. Asking for a ticket out of hell felt as absurd as it sounded when he heard himself say it.

~

Still in shock, Paul boarded the flight en route to Hawaii to meet his fiancée. The attendant checked his boarding pass against the manifest. The name matched his ticket. It looked like him. But it wasn't.

None of it felt real. His fiancée's perfume. The doll-like perfection of the hotel concierge. The cool ocean breeze wafting through the lobby. The rich aroma of roasted Kona coffee and fresh flowers. Light switches and flush toilets. Clean clothes. Ice. He had never noticed the miracle of any of it before the war.

He climbed between the starched white sheets and felt her radiant warmth. He hesitated to close his eyes, fearing he would wake up, soaking wet and shivering in the darkness on the jungle floor.

He assured himself that he had left the war behind, if only for a while, but his mind couldn't buy the empty promise of safety. So, it stayed in the jungle while the world assaulted his senses.

Civilization brought too much of everything: too much movement. Too much noise. Too many smells. Too many strangers. Too many doors and corners he couldn't see through or around. He strained to follow everything as if his life depended on it because what seemed like only moments ago, it had.

In spite of a world of luxuries unimaginable hours earlier, Paul didn't want to go anywhere. He didn't want to do anything. He couldn't bring himself to enjoy the freedom to indulge his every long-suppressed want. Like a man suddenly released from bondage, the glut of abundance choked him.

Paul spent his reward of a week with the love of his life in a Hawaiian paradise in his room, engulfed in anxiety. Looks of concern only added to his shame. A nauseating truth set in; though he survived the savagery of the war by dreaming of returning home to her, he no longer knew this world.

He just needed some rest, he told her. He was telling himself some version of that same story—selling hollow assurances while he bought time to figure out the man staring back at him in the hotel mirror.

When he was in the bush, all he could dream of was getting back to the world. Now that he was out, all he could think about was the inevitability of going back. That's why he couldn't let this alien world dull his sensibilities.

No. He couldn't get soft.

Not now. Not ever.

Paul saw what happened to those who gave up—the half-steppers, those that lost their edge. Those who couldn't stop dreaming of returning to this world. Or those who became complacent and surrendered to their misery. To their exhaustion. To their hopelessness.

They no longer had the energy or the will to heed their heightened senses. They no longer heard the clamor of their equipment in the bush. Or watched where they planted their next footstep. They no longer cupped the cherry of their cigarette at night. Some were simply beyond caring.

No. Paul *was* going to make it back to her.

He didn't have the words to explain to her how he became that stranger in the mirror. He didn't yet understand it himself. That would have to wait. For decades.

He couldn't describe what being hunted by every creature in the jungle did to him—they all wanted to devour him for coming to their country. They didn't know it wasn't of his choosing. They didn't care. They only knew he was not of their land.

Paul couldn't leave it to chance. Scared or not, he had to decide if he was going to survive … or not. He *would* make it home to her.

He reflected on the Huey's colored smoke trail that led the way back. He fulfilled all that was asked of him. And it was a lot. The government demanded twelve months in Vietnam. It was an impossibly long year that changed everything. Paul decided there was only one way out. He chose courage—he was scared and did it anyway. But no one told him that the war would cling to him for a lifetime.

It visited him at night when he could sleep. When he couldn't, he stood vigil in the darkness with his eyes trained on the front door.

Scared to make a sound.

Waiting for anything. Waiting for everything.

Waiting for the hunters to come.

⟋⟍⟍⟋

Epilogue: To this day, Paul sleeps on his couch in the living room in full view of his front door with protection near at hand. Even then, sound rest is hard to come by. His greatest priority remains protecting himself and his family. Though he's made gains in therapy, Paul continues to struggle with the fear the jungle instilled in him. He acknowledges that the legacy of Vietnam remains with him, in some way, on a daily basis. While I wish I could bring a well-deserved peace to all of my patients, sometimes this does not come in the form of significant or lasting symptomatic relief.

8

Unlucky Strikes

He knew better than to tell her why he couldn't sleep last night. It didn't keep his wife from asking, but the answer of "Vietnam" stopped the conversation—it always did.

When Allen told his PTSD group he was up most of the night, they offered a safer space to bring up the reasons. For a moment, he dangled the truth he didn't dare share with his wife. But he wasn't ready to go there yet. As the group leader, I looked for a path to help him tell the truth that he couldn't at home.

"And that's what kept you up all night thinking about Vietnam— things in *general*?"

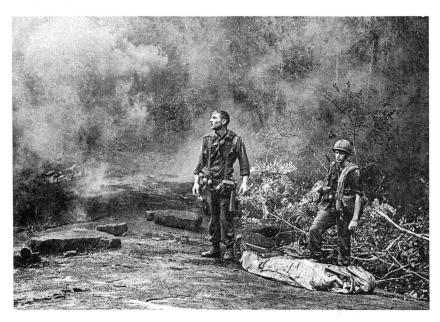

KIA in body bag waiting for extraction, 503rd Inf, 173 AB, National Archives.

I studied his face as he contemplated the invitation to tell us the real reason behind his insomnia, but he was still reluctant. Allen needed to go to where it hurt, but it was going to be his way.

For him, the war was mostly confined to the small 19th combat engineers base wedged between the South China Sea and the mountains of the Central Highlands in Vietnam. This thinly defended base relied on the larger infantry bases surrounding it for its security.

This area of operations was also a VC stronghold, and the enemy took every opportunity to remind them that America was unwelcome in their backyard. Attacks came regularly and daily life on the vulnerable base orbited around surviving the next one.

He sat looking at the floor and considering the offer to revisit the tiny base that bulged of bad memories. The room waited in silence. He glanced at the clock and then back at the floor before starting to speak.

"Well, last night, I was thinking about body bags. Bags that would be lined up, waiting for the chopper to fly them out and on their way home." Those bags were the outer contours of the story, but he was still not sure he wanted to make it personal—personal hurt.

More silence.

"Last night, the bags you were thinking about … did you know the men in them?" I studied his reaction. He fidgeted with the magazine he brought into group, its cover photo competing with the image emerging in his head.

We were getting closer.

"See, in Vietnam, people got hurt and killed so often that it just became a part of daily life there. You could be bullshitting with someone in the morning and later that day, they'd be lying in one of those bags. You'd be talking to a guy about anything … like cigarettes."

"Cigarettes?" I echoed following his trail.

"Yeah … see, where I was, there was no PX, and no place to buy cigarettes. You had to trade for everything, and getting the right cigarettes, your brand, was a problem."

The standard World War II vintage C-ration box, their daily staple, contained four miserably stale cigarettes. After that, a guy was on his own. There was only one other place to get them in Allen's war—SP packs.

"SP" stood for "sundries pack" and was the Army's answer to supplying fielded-combat troops with luxuries that the rest of Americans back home took for granted. They contained soap, gum, shaving equipment, chewing tobacco, lighter flints, writing paper, toothbrushes, tooth powder, and "tropical" chocolate bars whose formula was designed to withstand the furnace-like heat of Southeast Asia.

For many soldiers in that war, the only way they could differentiate

Vietnam from hell was because their SP chocolate had not yet melted. Even some of the Vietnamese kids who begged near the bases wouldn't eat it.

By far, the most valuable items in the SP pack were the cartons of cigarettes it contained. The guys who didn't smoke took cigarettes because they could be traded for something of value. But for guys who smoked, whether you got your brand was of great concern. It was one of the few things a soldier could look forward to. When every day might be your last, this small comfort might be the most important last thing one could do.

A guy's luck depended on where he was when the SPs arrived, where it was opened, and who got there ahead of you. If you were outside the wire, you were fortunate if you had a buddy looking out for your interests or if you received anything at all. In the desperate search for your preferred pack of smokes, you had to find the GIs who beat you there. Then the negotiations would begin. And that was how Allen met Greg.

"In Vietnam, we went by last names or nicknames. I remember Greg simply because he got a lot of mail. I hardly got any mail while I was in Vietnam, so that stood out to me. I'd hear his name yelled at mail call."

As first light broke, Allen and Greg were on guard duty. They were working a deal. Greg unloaded the resupply truck yesterday so he got first dibs on the SP. Now he had a carton of Lucky Strikes for sale.

Soldiers in war need something to hold on to. Allen saw too many body bags stacked by that helipad. Earlier that day, the men in those bags were dreaming of a better life—the car they fantasized about, some combat pay in their pocket and, if they were lucky, a girl and maybe a job waiting back home. Wishing for anything in the bush was chancy. Some dared not dream because death was always waiting. The dreams of the men in those bags were over.

But cigarettes … well … you could almost count on them.

The negotiation took but a minute. Luckys were in high demand, so it cost Allen the carton he didn't want plus an additional 500 piasters. He didn't mind the premium—it was that or menthols, and he hated those.

It gave him something to look forward to and that was a hard thing to come by at any price in Vietnam. "What's an extra 500 pi?" he asked himself as he conjured lighting up his first one only hours from now. Besides, money was for men with a future.

A rosy dawn spread through the concertina as they shook hands. They had terms but the deal would have to wait. Greg was on the routine morning mine sweeping duty of Highway 1. In the distance, Allen heard the quad fifty "black widow" fire up its diesel engine to prepare for its security escort mission.

The awesome firepower of its four .50 caliber M2 machine guns was feared by all. Allen quietly upped the odds of his getting his Luckys after Greg's team came back in. No one fucked with the black widow.

It was Allen's turn to stay in the wire. While this improved his chances of surviving another day, the price was the drudgery of base duty.

According to his superiors, there was always work for a soldier to do; bunkers needed construction, the parapet required reinforcement, and equipment was always in need of repair. The oppressive heat and humidity only added to the misery, as the pasty mix of sweat, salt, and red laterite dust of the earth caked sunburnt skin.

Every soldier looked to alleviate their suffering and square themselves away for another day of staying alive. While Allen was designated "US" (draftee), he figured that if he had to be there, he would simply do what needed to be done until he didn't have to anymore. By staying busy and surviving until the next sunrise, he was one day closer to leaving this God-forsaken place. But today, he had something to look forward to. By nightfall, he'd have his cigarettes. This thought helped pass the time.

Others addressed their suffering not by working, but by complaining about working. One of the Spec 4s in Allen's work detail that day was a skinny kid from the streets of Philadelphia. His name was Marcus. According to Allen, he had a high-pitched voice and bitched about everything. He only remembered his first name because he was so annoying.

Marcus also talked about politics. He would point out that Vietnam was a white man's war and that he was in the wrong place. In contrast to Allen's "US" status, Marcus was RA ("regular army")—a volunteer. In Allen's book, *he* was the one who should never have been there, and the painful irony made him all the more resentful of Marcus's incessant complaints.

Yet others simply suffered silently. The third guy in the work detail was a muscular Puerto Rican kid who never said a word to anyone. Rumor was that he had stabbed someone back home and the judge gave him the choice of prison or Vietnam. Though he never spoke, the guys in the unit couldn't help but to wonder if he now regretted that decision.

However, his past was of no concern to Allen; the big Puerto Rican simply nodded and did what he was told to do. As the highest-ranking man, this made Allen's life just a little bit easier. It freed his mind to look forward to the end of the day when Greg's road-clearing detail would return. They all worked side by side in silence while Marcus continued to complain to an invisible, unsympathetic audience.

The work wore on as the midday sun beat down upon them. As they toiled, sounds of combat intermittently played in the background. The war was always there—sometimes farther, sometimes closer. Then the next exchange of erratic gunfire sounded a little closer than was typical.

Allen had been in Vietnam for many months now. His hearing and ability to locate sounds sharpened along with the rest of his survival senses. His ears perked and strained to decipher the message of incoming echoes. While there was no immediate threat to him, its signature was unsettling—it was coming from the highway.

The numbness that set in among soldiers was a blessing and a curse. Which one it turned out to be didn't seem to be up to the man, but controlled by something beyond him. When their body wouldn't block the fear or pain, they found anesthesia wherever they could.

There were the beer rations, but hot brew did little to quench their thirst or their pain. While the locals peddled drugs, other times they found relief from the medics. The potent propoxyphene ampules buried in the widely available Darvon capsules were particularly prized. When it couldn't come from chemicals, the men created mantras they repeated often enough that one came to believe it.

"Yeah … it don't mean nuthin'—not a thing."

But all too often, it *did* mean something.

Sometimes, those black bags laying by the chopper pad contained men that used to be your friends. Other times, they contained people you knew from your outfit, but didn't know well. And sometimes, they contained men you knew by their first name only because they got a lot of mail.

That day, Allen knew one man in a body bag. He was eagerly awaiting his return from duty so he could trade him a carton and 500 piasters for those Luckys.

The group listened as Allen somberly reflected on the real reason he couldn't sleep last night. It had not been something general—it was quite specific. And it was not the end of his war story. It was just another day of trying to stay alive in Vietnam.

But on that particular day, it meant *something*.

"How come it was always the good ones who got killed?" Allen rhetorically asked.

The other veterans in the group quietly scrolled through their own lists of all the good ones they knew who never returned home. They pictured the faces of men they sometimes knew for weeks, days, or hours before being killed, only to disappear into a rolled poncho or a black bag, never to be spoken of again.

There was no answer to his question.

There was only another sleepless night remembering a good kid who got a lot of mail and happened to have had a carton of Allen's favorite brand of cigarettes.

Epilogue: Many group therapy sessions concluded because we ran out of time to find some resolution. Others, like this one, ended without resolution because there was none to be had. Men serving closely together in war often form enduring bonds stronger than family. However, death's randomness and omnipresent threat undermines the herd instinct of those in combat to seek physical and emotional safety in one another. Many soldiers protect themselves from the horror and death and loss of one another by avoiding close bonds. Allen's story speaks to these fickle connections shared between soldiers who co-exist in a combat zone, often acquainted by mere proximity or happenstance. While such relationships were often fleeting, the trauma surrounding their rupture can, and often does, persist as it has for Allen.

9

The Tent

He didn't plan on talking about it again today. As he started off the session's dialogue, he wasn't aware when he walked into his PTSD group, he would be going back to the worst place he had ever been.

A new resident co-leader introduced herself to the group, and as he tried to commit the new resident's name to memory, Jeff scrolled through students he'd seen come and go. The first co-leader he met after joining the group bestowed upon him the "Cocksucker award."

At the time, Jeff accepted that curious accolade with a laugh and even pride, but it now produced more serious reflection—clearly, this

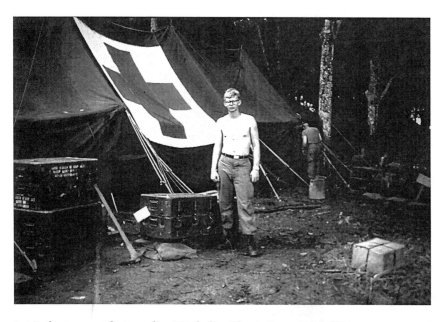

1st Infantry combat medic, Michelin Plantation, 1966 (Veteran personal photograph).

unconventional nomination required some explanation. He sheepishly turned to directly address the new resident.

"The reason I got that award was that when I first joined the group, well.... I was in sad shape. I was so angry. Every time I opened my mouth to speak, that word came out of my mouth ... usually because of my rage at the military and political leadership whom I blamed for decades for what happened in Vietnam ... for all those young men who were needlessly sacrificed. As I sit here now, I am realizing I have not used that word in a long time. The anger is not there like it used to be."

After that anger dissolved, he was surprised to encounter the feelings it camouflaged. And as he described to us how he vanquished his rage and the found his deep sadness waiting on the other side of it, it showed up once again.

Jeff halted in mid-sentence to fight the torrent rising up his throat. The redness beneath his eyes fanned out as facial muscles contracted to fight what was coming. He momentarily held his breath, spasmed in a sharp gasp, then surrendered. Desperately needed oxygen and the sadness waiting right behind it radiated throughout his body.

Jeff had been here before. This time, he let the tears flow. He now understood the anger was a clever distraction. He knew it was really about his grief and bearing witness, in gruesome detail, to the loss of life as a medic with the 1st Infantry Division at a forward aid station somewhere near the Michelin Rubber Plantation in III Corps in 1966. He just wasn't sure he could go back there now.

The grief also obscured the details. He knew only this: At some point during his tour in Vietnam, the 2/16th Infantry had a vicious battle with the Viet Cong. The wounded and dead poured off of the battlefield near his aid station. They were unprepared for the wave of casualties, and it quickly overwhelmed the veteran's small medical unit responsible for their first-line care.

Attached to that aid station, Jeff occupied, by himself, a small blacked-out canvas tent containing his field lab equipment, which he feverishly used to assist in the emergency care of those wounded. And in the back of that tent, in the sweltering jungle heat and humidity, was a growing pile of black bags holding the mangled bodies of the dead.

Because of that pile of bags, Jeff struggled to avoid anything that brought back the sickly-sweet stench of death. But wherever he went, the war found him.

As an avid outdoorsman, he would return from a hunting or fishing trip only to report his adventure derailed by some reminder of that tent. Idyllic trout streams were interrupted by the wafting odor of a decomposing animal. Camping under the stars in his tent stirred vivid nightmares of the bodies of the dead crowding him as he slept.

"That tent is my nightmare. It is where my main problems from the war come from," he whispered with haunted, bloodshot eyes.

The group rallied around Jeff as he stood at the chasm of his grief. He knew they would hold the emotional belay that would prevent him from falling into the bottomless hole of the war—a hole that every man in the room feared disappearing into and not being able to find their way back. But every time a group member stood at its edge, it tested the bonds of trust among them.

"I didn't plan on going here today, Doc," Jeff half-stated, half-pleaded.

"It's your call," I assured him. A merciful and respectful silence filled the room.

The group took the extended pause as a signal for help and swooped in. They let Jeff contemplate the choice while they tossed around what they had learned about emotional healing, the role of constructing the details of their combat tours, and the critical ingredient of communalizing the trauma within this sacred circle of listeners. This went for some time before I glanced at the ticking clock—it beckoned a ruling. I turned back to Jeff with the invitation.

"I wanted to make sure that you have time to get back there with us if that is indeed what you want for yourself."

Tears were already flowing down his cheeks. "I wasn't sure we were going to have enough ... enough time." He centered himself in the chair and planted both feet squarely on the floor. The group steadied for the descent back into the abyss.

Jeff brought us back to the disorientation of an event with few external markers of time and space; that tent became the scene of his nightmares had no exact locators—there was no date, no day, no specific location. He didn't have the name of the ones they triaged, stabilized, and sent to the better equipped medical evacuation facilities. And, most importantly to him, he didn't have the names of the dead.

"All I can tell you is that we were in or around the Michelin Rubber Plantation and that it was 1966. And that I was alone."

But it wasn't just the details he didn't know or forgot. It was the ones he couldn't forget—the sensory memories that lived within him in an un-ending present. Through the tears, he described the overwhelming sense of grief, the stifling heat, and the way the suffocating odors of the dead mixed with the oppressive humidity and dank background of heavily mildewed canvas.

"It was unbelievable...," he whispered.

As Jeff relived those putrid smells, faces in the group room instinctively contorted. Noses wrinkled, evading the invisible stink now assaulting them. They found their own haunting memories attached to that unforgettable odor. To a man, every set of eyes were now trained on the blank screen of the laminate floor tiles watching their own version of the horror show. Playing today was the fragility of life, the taint of death, and the perfidy of men in war.

The group flowed that day, but not because anyone, including me, knew the right thing to say. It flowed because we *didn't* have the right words. The sensorium-driven story defied language, producing a spontaneous dialogue that was more emotionally raw and real than any of us planned on contemplating that day. I can remember almost nothing of what was actually said and more of *how* it was said as a palpable reverence filled the room.

The veterans encircled their ailing brother, created sacred space, and tended to him. They honored the unidentified dead in the tent, and Jeff for carrying their memories. They created something that Jeff had not received in the last five decades—witnesses to help him grieve the nameless dead, acknowledge the steep cost of his duties, and a safe place to touch the places that hurt.

And touch them he did. But this time, when Jeff saw the body bags, fought the next breath of putrid air, and salved his wounded soul, he didn't do it in that tent alone.

Epilogue: For decades, Jeff's staunch avoidance kept his symptoms associated with that medical tent fragmented and unintegrated, contributing to his persistent and painful intrusions of this trauma. In keeping with our model of recovery, Jeff confronted his past, researched the events associated with this battle, completed his trauma narrative, and communalized it in group.

Jeff eventually discovered this nameless, timeless memory recounted the battle of Courtenay Plantation near the village of Xa Cam My on April 11–12, 1966. During that battle, the 2/16th Infantry, 1st Infantry Division, sought to draw out the Viet Cong D800 battalion and were ambushed. American forces suffered seventy wounded and thirty-seven killed, with Charlie company taking eighty percent casualties. One of the KIAs included an Air Force pararescue man, Airman 1st Class William Pitsenbarger, Jr., who was posthumously awarded the Medal of Honor for his heroic actions portrayed in the 2019 movie *The Last Full Measure*. In the process of researching this battle, Jeff discovered the names of those thirty-seven soldiers killed, some of whom filled the body bags in his tent. The men who gave their lives in this battle during Operation Abilene are honored on the Vietnam Memorial Wall on Panel 06E, lines 97–105.

10

The Low Side

Though his hearing was not what it used to be, Eric's ears perked at the unmistakable blade thump in the distance—nothing sounds like a Huey.

The restored 1971 Bell UH-1 Iroquois "Huey" chopper was inbound. The anticipation coursed through my body with its approach. I was waiting for a ride in this vintage warbird that would bring me ever closer to the Vietnam veterans I care for. I wanted to feel something of what they encountered as they were carried into battle, even if my flight was in Perryville, Missouri, at the Missouri National Veterans Memorial, and no one was shooting at me. However, this first ride was special because I went to the newly constructed Wall that day for its grand opening with Eric.

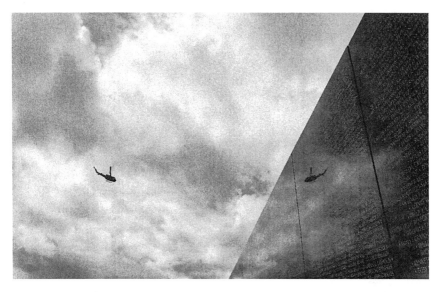

Huey reflection in "the Wall" at Missouri's National Veterans Memorial (author collection).

I met Eric at Channel Nine, our local St. Louis PBS affiliate. Because of my experience as a VA combat trauma psychologist, I was invited to be a member of a panel discussion with him following a screening of the documentary *Take Me Home Huey*.

Eric was on this panel because the film was about him and the crew of his medevac chopper, their combat service in Vietnam, and the tragic crash that forever bound them together. Forty-five years later, an artist and a group of invested war vets found the rotting fuselage of their helicopter in an Arizona junkyard. They restored and transformed it into a work of art to raise awareness of combat veterans' struggles with Post-Traumatic Stress Disorder.

As their project progressed, they researched the aircraft's history using its serial number, #174, and traced it to the men who fought and died in it during the war. In the process of shooting the film, the traumatized survivors of that medevac crew were serendipitously reunited, and their trauma, pain and healing process intimately shared with us on screen.

The restored Huey emerged against the billowing cumulus and approached the group of us anxiously awaiting its arrival. I was the first in line and had my pick of any seat. They were flying with the doors open. I craved the thrill so many Huey door gunners described, so when the safety briefing officer began planning seating assignments, the decision was easy—I chose the gun well. I would share that now-unarmed, but cramped seat with a vet who served with the 5th Mechanized Infantry in 1969—a ground pounder. I was surprised to hear this helicopter ride was on his bucket list too. Though in Vietnam for a full tour, he never flew in a Huey. My pulse quickened as the faint sound and the dark speck in the sky grew.

The echoes enveloped us as the blades beat the heavy cloud-filled air. Whoop.... Whoop.... Whoop.... Whoop!

The Huey flared for landing. The brilliant emerald grass submitted in pulsing concentric waves as the rotor wash pressed into the LZ. It gently touched down in the shortly cropped field and brought with it a living portrait of the Vietnam War.

As the whirling blades slowed to idle, a time-traveler—an olive drab flight suit-clad warrior—emerged from the ship's thorax. The smoked visor of the Gentex flight helmet concealed most of his features save for his gray mustache partially obscured by his coms-microphone.

Though anonymous, Eric didn't need to see his face to feel the connection; the details of his uniform told his story. On his left breast were his flight wings. His right shoulder bore his combat patch—the silhouetted black horse bust against the divided yellow field signaled they were brothers—1st Cavalry, Airmobile.

With this crew chief's beckoning wave, it was time to load the first group. As I stood, Eric leaned in close to overcome the whirling rotors.

"If you go down, go out the high side ... not the low side."

He said it with a wry smile, but his advice came from a place of experience, wisdom, and pain. And he would have known. Fifty years ago, Eric was pilot of a Huey not unlike the one I was about to board. He served with the 15th Medical Battalion of the 1st Cavalry in Vietnam in 1968–69. He didn't need to go on a Huey ride—he had been in one more times than he could count.

As I came to know Eric, he shared more of his captivating war history. He was drafted in 1965 and, while he wished to serve, he concluded early in his military enlistment that he did not want the burden of killing. Flying appealed to him, and that ambition and his moral apprehension steered him towards medical evacuation. He would fly out the wounded and, in so doing, serve by saving lives instead of taking them. Near the top of his flight school class, he went to gun-ship training just before graduation from flight school. Just days before shipping to Ft. Sam Houston to complete his medevac training, the calendar intervened—it was late January 1968.

The shock of the Tet Offensive changed everything. Due to the soaring casualties, Eric's entire flight class was sent straight to Vietnam. The Army needed helicopter pilots—quickly. Like many other young men rushed through the training process, Eric would just have to figure out the medevac part. Though he was committed to sticking to his plan, the Army needed him elsewhere. He was sent to B Troop, 1/9th, 1st Air Cavalry.

Though short-lived, Eric started this initial assignment as the outgoing troop commander's pilot—until his replacement arrived. The incoming Major was an archetypal warrior and real-life model for the bulletproof fictional character, Colonel Kilgore, in Coppola's *Apocalypse Now*. As Martin Sheen narrates in that film, "the 1st of the 9th, an old cavalry unit, had cashed in their horses for helicopters and went tear-assing around Vietnam looking for the shit." This new commanding officer had no patience for soldiers unwilling to support his aggressive mission—killing as many of the enemy as possible. Eric lasted three days as his co-pilot flying a C Model Huey gunship.

His demand for a transfer out of this storied outfit was incomprehensible to leadership and quietly ushered through to avoid the tarnish of embarrassment. Eric was transferred to the 15th Medical Battalion where he served with distinction as a medevac chopper pilot for the last eight months of his tour.

During that stint, his crew received a casualty pick-up call for a downed scout ship. On the horn was Co. B, 1st of the 9th. Eric was in communication via radio with the commander and brought his Huey to participate in the evacuation. When that officer learned who was piloting the bird that came in under fire to get his men out, he questioned, "Is that *you*, Berla?!?"

Eric simply replied, "Yes, sir."

"I was wrong about you." the Major offered in a rare admission. He later backed this apology with recognition and honor. Eric was awarded the Distinguished Flying Cross for coming to B Troop's aide during that engagement.

In February of 1969, Eric returned home at the end of his tour. While he was stateside, on Valentine's Day, #174 flew a medevac mission in Binh Long province and was shot down by enemy forces. The aircraft went down hard, collapsing the left skid and altering the angle of the whirling rotors.

When it crashed, SP4 Gary Dubach, the crew chief, leapt out of the low side of the aircraft with his machine gun to establish a defensive position, but fell. SP4 Stephen Schumacher, the medic, followed him to render aid. The wounded warbird's now-tilted rotor blades killed them both.

The surviving crew struggled with the deaths of Gary and Stephen in their own way. *Take Me Home Huey* told the story of #174's transformation from warbird to memorial art, but the heart of the film was the healing of the men traumatized by the loss of their brothers. That they died on Valentine's Day forever welded together love and loss.

After my unforgettable Huey ride, Eric and I approached the black granite memorial wall. An unspoken agreement of respectful silence and organic solitude set in. We each had two names to find. We each had our reasons for finding them. We went to find his first.

The captivating power of the Wall grew as we approached its nadir. The seemingly infinite names blurred as we walked. That blur hid the individuals but accentuated the many. I became painfully conscious of the obvious—so many names.

So many sons, brothers, husbands, and fathers. So many.

As we approached panel 32W, our pace slowed, and the blur of humanity became more distinct and emotionally incisive. Even with the panel and line numbers in hand, the search among the thousands of dead was dizzying. Eric stood in silence, transfixed and searching.

The feelings welled up from my core. I stood behind him grieving for men I had never met, and only knew through Eric and the film that brought us together. I was watching for the moment he would discover their etched names, not knowing what that connection might bring. This was not a process to rush; one could never be sure what emotion the Wall may pull from a man, what pocket of hurt it may find, what wound it may touch.

Without a word passing between us, I sensed that my eyes were needed. I started scanning the rows, the sameness of their form slurring my methodical effort. Frustrated, my instincts took over and it was not long before slamming into the name as if I had suddenly reached the end of an unforgiving tether.

"DUBACH."

Momentarily stunned by finding this single man in a sea of men, my eyes reversed slowly for confirmation.

"GARY L."

Then they blurred again as they filled with tears. I took a moment to let the wave within me crest, and then looked over to see him still scanning.

"Eric ... here they are."

It took a few more moments to find his medic, Stephen L. Schumacher. He was listed three lines down, but with many names separating these two fallen brothers in arms. The solemnity of that discovery came with its own painful realization; the surviving crew of #174 was joined by many other American families for whom Valentine's Day would never be the same.

As we stood paying silent homage, the airborne Huey continued to circle above us as if flying top cover for their lost brethren. Eric couldn't help but to track its path as its reassuring signature echoed off the Wall. Looking at a few still photographs I took of those moments later revealed a haunting image of the banking Huey against a cloud filled sky, its ghosted reflection captured in the Wall's granite face.

That picture flawlessly captured the richness of the day and the nexus of its many connections: it embodied Eric's connection to his history, my connection to him, and the collective grief we both carry connected to the war in Vietnam for our own reasons.

It also captured the pact set in stone I have made with these veterans, and them with me; they have honored me with their trust, their stories, and the painful lessons of their venture through the underworld of war.

And as I took my seat in the gun well and buckled myself into the Huey, I understood the value of what Eric shared that day at the Wall, and tucked away the dark wisdom he had passed down to me. The rhythmic idle of the blades broke into a smooth acceleration. Eric smiled and gave a thumbs-up as he raised his camera to shoot our lift-off.

"Yes ... the high side ... never the low side."

11

Forged in the Jungle

For a fisherman, it was the trip of a lifetime. He and his best friend had long been planning an adventure to the pristine Canadian lake on a protected Native Indian reservation. Reachable only by bush plane, its virgin wilderness promised the remote sanctuary and elusive peace they were seeking.

For fifty years to be exact.

As their departure date approached, Don's body and his mind were escalating their silent, visceral protest. His nerves had his stomach in knots, his GI tract was in distress, and his wife noticed their increasingly edgy conversations. When she finally asked if he still wanted to go through with the trip, a yet unspoken and pressurized truth escaped, surprising them both.

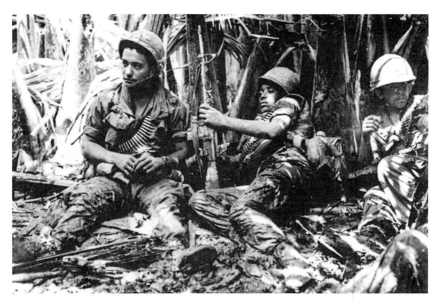

U.S. Army troops take break in jungle while on patrol, National Archives, by Sp4 Dennis Kurpius.

"I'm not sure I want to go, OK?!"

Don sat in my office trying to sort out what was happening to him as the departure date approached.

On the surface, there were the uncertainties of the plan. Don and Garitt had been fishing together before, but this would be the first time they would do so for seventeen days, alone in a lake cabin in the middle of nowhere. Don assuaged his wife's concerns with a rented satellite phone for emergencies. But that was her fear, not his. He worried what they may find in their isolation when revisiting the darkness of their shared past.

～

Don and Garitt met at Ft. Ord, California, for advanced individual training (AIT). It was their last stop before deploying to Vietnam. They bonded quickly as they were mid-westerners and both assigned a MOS of 11C; these teenagers, who were destined for lifelong friendship, would soon become mortar men in the infantry.

Their Drill Instructor at Ft. Ord had eight weeks to ready them for war, and he prepared Don and Garitt's training platoon as best he could. He was a decent and caring man who only partially concealed that truth with his hardened authoritarianism required for the job. Not that he would ever have admitted it, but under the theatrical yelling, his heart quietly ached. He knew where these young warriors were going. And he knew they wouldn't all be coming back. He felt he owed them the truth and, at the end of every training cycle, he prepared his men to hear it.

To celebrate Don and Garitt's graduation from AIT, the Drill Sergeant bought the unit beer and they all got drunk. Then he told those young men the reality of where they were going.

"He told us thirty percent of us were going to get hit and what percentage of us were never coming home. He said those of us that survived would never be the same. Either way, we were *all* going to be wounded by the war."

Don paused, his eyes and voice signaling that he was reliving the macabre briefing. The fear of the inescapable set seeds of dread in them all. However, in a war filled with lies, there was also a profound appreciation that someone cared enough to tell them the hard truth.

"He told us that when we got over there, the most important thing we could do to improve our odds of surviving was to find an 'old guy' who could teach us what we needed to know." Don did not forget this parting advice.

When he got to Vietnam, the Army allocated the fresh arrivals by the cold arithmetic of need. How he and Garitt stayed together was blind luck as they were pitilessly split off from the rest of the arriving replacements from Ft. Ord. Before they grasped their vague instructions, they were herded onto a Huey with several others in freshly issued gear, its newness attesting to the final moments of innocence of the men wearing it.

As the chopper headed north towards II Corps, the young soldiers tried to stifle their fear as they were delivered into the jaws of the war. Don and Garitt sat in frozen silence, staring at the deceptive beauty of the dense emerald mat far beneath their dangling jungle boots.

But at least they were together.

As the Huey leapfrogged from one firebase to the next, Don gathered information on their fate—anything to fill the sickening void of uncertainty. At each base, some troops offered empty assurances. Others wore weary faces too tired to muster pity. But with each stop, the signs worsened. Don recounted the mounting terror instilled by the weathered soothsayers.

"Every time we got ready for the next leg of the journey, they would say, 'you'll be ok as long as they don't take you to the Central Highlands.' And that's where we went. Then they said, don't worry…. You'll probably be fine as long as you don't go to Pleiku. Then we landed in Pleiku. Then, they said, just pray you're not going to Đắk Tô … and then we arrived in Đắk Tô."

The name meant nothing to Don and Garritt. That changed quickly.

His eyes widened as he continued narrating his first day in the bush. "Đắk Tô … It was there we discovered we were going to Hill 1338. That's when they told us … that on that hill … a lot of our guys had been….

…had been slaughtered…."

His voice started shaking as he relived the Huey's approach into their final stop.

The low hanging clouds misted the highlands, creating a pillowy but foreboding shroud obscuring their nearing destination. The fog gradually gave way to the dense top-growth jungle below the descending chopper. Then, out of nowhere, appeared the jarring, pocked moonscape of 1338. An apocalypse of chewed earth, shattered and charred tree trunks, and debris of past battles smothered the dead hilltop.

After the grievous loss of American life on that hill, it was mercilessly bombed and napalmed to lifelessness. Like ants, olive clad men dug through the earth to create a fortress network of slit trenches, concertina wire, and reinforced bunkers. Near that hill was a highly contested bridge defended by mortar positions and dug in infantry. As Don described the scene, it became clear why he was brought to this cursed place. As a replacement mortar man, Don had finally arrived at his first combat duty station.

The Huey's blades powered down as the veteran NCO at the LZ

instructed the nervous replacements to dismount and line up. The Sergeant was a lifer—an "old guy." He addressed the row of wide-eyed soldiers standing at stiff attention in front of him.

"I'm looking for three men … impress me!"

Don remembered the life-saving advice at Ft. Ord. The Sergeant stopped in front of Don, his penetrating glare X-raying his soul. This was his chance.

"Where you from, Soldier?"

"St. Louis, sir!"

Don didn't know it yet, but he had just found his "old guy."

The Sarge hailed from the north side of the city, but he didn't let on to that just yet. He was looking for a few good men, and *he* was the one doing the interviewing.

Don stumbled through the barrage of questions trying to decode the right answers. Some felt forged to fail his candidacy, only to find follow-up queries that lead him through doors he wasn't sure he should be walking through.

"You smoke marijuana, soldier?" Sarge asked.

"No, sir!"

"You've *never* smoked weed?" The door slowly creaked open.

"Well, ur…. I mean, sir…. I've *tried* it … but I would never smoke on duty, sir!"

"*Never?*"

Sarge's questions wrapped around Don like the tightening coils of a boa, looking to squeeze out a truth he could count on or suffocate him trying. But Sarge had to know. Most replacements weren't worth the trouble and they died like flies because they hadn't yet learned what it took to survive.

In the jungle, one couldn't count on much except the guy next to you; a man needed to know who was sharing his foxhole. The Sarge's style, authority, and search for reliable men of lower rank hid dark incentives that would reveal themselves in due time.

After Sarge completed Don's interview, he asked one last question about the stiffened replacements toeing the line with him. He had but one recommendation. And that's how Don and Garitt wound up sharing not only a foxhole and the hell of Vietnam, but a lifetime of friendship.

"Okay…. You … you … and you … step forward," Sarge commanded.

Don passed. And that night, in the jungles of Đắk Tô, overlooking a bridge, his Sergeant and newly discovered "old guy," christened his adoption and got him high.

Sarge was a natural. After Don latched onto his "old guy," he taught him and Garitt how to survive in the bush. He groomed their combat gunnery skills and the art of indirect fire in guerrilla warfare. They learned well, and for that they continued to live, while many others didn't.

Sometimes it was their hard-fought wisdom. Sometimes it was simply the odds—a fortune that Don still couldn't figure out if he deserved while so many others' luck had run out.

But some weren't going to bet on chance to make it out. And that was the Faustian bargain that Don and Garitt unknowingly signed on to. While Sarge turned them into skilled jungle fighters, there were a few tricks about surviving that he kept to himself.

One of those was finding the right men to do the job, so he didn't have to. Sarge was going to make it out of this place alive—no matter what.

At first, his men were blinded by the light of idolatry that shone upon Sarge. That gave way to his enviable knack for knowing how to catch the rare breaks the war grudgingly offered up. But that facade soon began to crumble. Endless patrols through the jungle will do that.

Don's unit hacked their way through the impenetrable brush and humped the punishing terrain, eventually finding their destined way point. They would collapse into an exhausted heap of men and equipment covered with the sweat and grime they had just earned. Shortly thereafter, a helicopter would land near their position, and the Sarge would jump out, appearing fresh and shouting orders.

In the bush, one became wise quickly. Seeing the stark truth in a situation was the surest way of surviving it. It didn't take long to recognize that he just wasn't catching breaks.

No. The Sarge made his own luck and used his rank to manufacture it. Among the men, reverence faded into simmering resentment.

But it had never killed anyone. At least not yet.

They weren't supposed to be in Laos and Cambodia at this point in the war, but they were. The 4th Infantry was hunting the NVA who used their neighboring country's neutrality as a sanctuary from which to conduct operations against South Vietnam.

The U.S. military was growing impatient with their politicians. Elements of the 4th Infantry Division were covertly pivoting to the west. However, it would be another year until the government allowed the U.S. Army to officially invade Cambodia.

And that was part of Don's problem—they weren't supposed to be in Cambodia so according to the military, they weren't. At least not on paper.

Decades later, when Don made inquiries into the military archives to find out where his unit had been in Cambodia, and the many men they lost, he could find nothing to corroborate what happened there. He had only the reluctant testimony of he and Garitt's partially excavated hellish memories.

Don didn't want to revisit that push into Cambodia in a therapy session or in a backcountry cabin in the Canadian wilderness. He and Garitt held interlocking pieces of their secret. They could hardly stand to talk about it, but the truth was impossible to avoid for long. They tried many times over the years, but the amount of alcohol required for that journey towards the pain lead to either arguments, a numb stupor, or both.

Don also tried on his own, assembling the jagged pieces of what happened the night elements of the 4th Infantry were massacred somewhere in the mountains of Cambodia. Frustrated with the stonewalling from a local government records center, he planned a trip to the Army's archives in Washington, D.C., in hopes of uncovering the truth. However, the terrorizing prospect of revisiting that place on his own brought on a mental collapse and required a respite psychiatric hospitalization to help reconstitute his mind.

He was vexed by his dilemma; he could neither approach the memory nor outrun it. And couldn't get past the betrayal. It now trapped him in life as it had on that unnumbered hill somewhere in Cambodia in 1969.

As was the often case in Vietnam, the decisions that sent men towards their deaths were far removed from the places they died. And it went all the way up the line. General officers were tired of being hamstrung by the politicians running the war from thousands of miles away. Field grade commanders were frustrated by the enemy's hit and run tactics, bleeding our military might one cut at a time.

Washington needed a victory, and that required more bodies to count. Though they were bombing North Vietnamese positions across the border for years, Cambodia remained officially neutral. Finally, leadership reached agreement—they planned to pursue the enemy into their Cambodian sanctuary. There they would find plenty of bodies to count.

Sarge had no plans on being counted. He saw too many young Americans leave Vietnam zipped up in bags. As his unit's column pushed west, he read the situation and sensed the narrow window rapidly closing. The slicks were coming en masse, ferrying in tons of ammo and supplies to feed the imminent push. Don's weary unit watched in disbelief as Sarge took the last supply chopper out, leaving his outfit leaderless. Now at the mercy of higher-ranking men who sat in safety, elements of the 4th pushed deep across the Cambodian border.

The first company that headed down the hill that night to make contact with the NVA unit waiting for them was cut to pieces. The bloodied remnants staggered back up the slope to their lines. But leadership wasn't going to let the enemy slip away. Don's company was next.

He and Garitt took a blood oath; they swore they would never reveal what happened—the secret of what they had to do to stay alive that night.

They took the horrifying scraps of that truth and buried them in the deepest hole they could find in their minds.

They neither saw nor heard from the Sarge ever again.

His betrayal welded the horror of that night in Cambodia into the most profound moral injury they would endure. It had fit the definition to a "T"; a betrayal of what's right, by leadership, in a high-stakes situation. It was also a destroyer of the fabled values that were drilled into them by the military, so the deceit went far above the rank of Sergeant.

Never leave a man behind. How many times were they told?

It started to test, then unravel much of the rest of it. In boot camp, they were methodically disassembled as civilians, and recast into men who would do the most unnatural of things. For each other. For their country. It was this very training that emboldened men to suppress their instinct to survive and follow orders, even into death.

But this truth, and the trust that cemented it into place, was one of many forgeries Don and Garitt would discover out there in the bush. Some men, both dead and alive, *were* left behind. And some men who swore otherwise left them there.

Don and Garitt tried to move on from the war. They each developed their ways of trying to forget, but that meant staying busy to the point of distraction, led to the bottom of a bottle, or both. Even then, the pain never stayed put for long.

They discovered the vexing problem with trauma and moral injury— you are okay until you're not. They could function as civilians when the pain stayed in its hole. However, it didn't take much. The hurt seeped in through the endless associations that wandered too close. Sometimes during the day, and most often at night.

There were times the images of the slaughter in Cambodia, and so many others they never thought they would survive, mingled into hellish nightmares. Like in country, they were grateful to see the rising sun, to live to see another day. But days, too, were fraught with unexpected trips back to the jungle. It came at any time and in so many ways.

A simple trip to the mall was the last place Don thought he'd find the war. But his daughter brought him over the jewelry counter to show him the golden crucifix she was eyeing. Suddenly, Don broke into a cold sweat as he relived the haunting memory of the panicked, overweight Sergeant who disappeared into the jungle in search of his heirloom cross he had lost on patrol and was never seen again.

Even a dream vacation could turn into a nightmare. Don and his wife were enjoying their Hawaiian adventure and day trip to the volcanic rainforest. He didn't notice it at first—he was too awestruck to catch it stalking him; the humidity, emerald foliage, filtered sunlight, scent of humus, and avian calls wafting through jungle. Suddenly, paradise transformed right before his eyes into the Vietnamese bush. In a panic, he cut that excursion short. Even decades later, the fear was right there waiting. For both of them.

While the two friends lived in the same city for many years, Don's retirement and his wife's work would take them a state away from Garitt. The miles stretched the elastic connection between the two men. When they were together, the unanswered questions about the war and their shared secrets tugged and tested them. Though they were betrayed, the jungle forged a bond of friendship that would never break.

⁓

The fishing boat rocked gently on the pristine, placid lake cloistered by the Canadian evergreens. The quiet was broken only by the soft rhythm of lapping waves against the hull. Words were unnecessary. The two lifelong friends sat in contented contemplation, watching their taut lines gradually disappearing into the infinite blueness.

12

Sleeping with the Dead

"Don't take away my hate, Doc. It's all I've got."

His solemn but stern eyes conveyed that serious truth. It wasn't quite a threat, but it wasn't a request either.

This man had been through hell. He had the right to hold onto whatever feelings he wanted to, even if he would pay a grievous price for it.

Harlan postured because I came too close—too close to the dark story he walled off inside of him thirty-nine years earlier. He shared his version

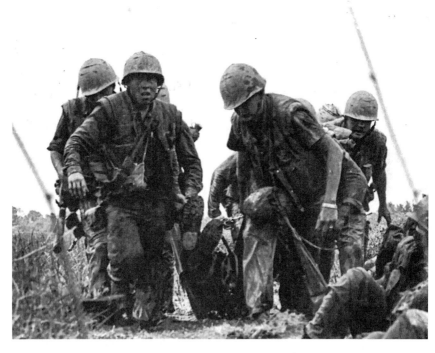

Marines carrying wounded to medevac, National Archives, USMC photograph A369791 by LCPL Curry.

of it with his PTSD therapy group once before, but today he steered out of the discussion. He didn't like where it was going.

The account he was willing to share gained the respect of his fellow Vietnam combat veterans because it described the day he earned the Silver Star. This valorous medal secured him a revered plot in Arlington Cemetery for when his time came. The group's collective respect was welcomed. The uninvited challenge of his version of what happened that day and his hatred towards those who betrayed him, however, was not.

But it was precisely this betrayal that was in question. Harlan blamed the three Marines in his fireteam who had violated their oath in the heat of battle. To him, that was the only perspective that mattered; they were fucking cowards and he couldn't hear otherwise.

It was simpler that way. They were the reason for all of it. All of his anger. All of his pain.

Harlan refused to see that his rage was greater than these three men. These Marines who in 1966 betrayed their motto, *Semper Fidelis,* were just his obvious targets.

There was plenty of blame to go around for the carnage. Some who should have been "always faithful," had been anything but. In Vietnam, it went all the way up the line to the White House. The decision makers took the same sworn oath Harlan did when he joined the Corps. He kept up his end. He expected everyone else to do the same.

Only they didn't.

And this is what his fellow group members wanted him to consider. They were convinced this misplaced rage was the linchpin between Harlan's angry head and his ailing heart.

It wasn't that his anger about the war was without justification. The group got it—they were mad about many of the same things he was. But they were also worried about Harlan's health—his anger was killing him.

For a man in his late fifties, his cardiologist was convinced that Harlan's prematurely advancing heart disease went beyond medical factors alone. At his last appointment, he was advised that he was speeding towards a heart attack. If he were to make progress on his concerning lab and test results, his chronic anger could no longer lie undisturbed.

Only he didn't want to hear that. Harlan wasn't one to bow to others simply because he was outvoted. It didn't matter how many initials one had after their surname. In fact, in his book, one's formal credentials were inversely related to one's credibility.

In Vietnam, those with impressive titles got a lot of good people killed. Harlan couldn't see how the decisions by men of high rank made their deaths any less of a waste. Even before the war, he was fervently independent and didn't take much for granted. No matter who the orders came from.

Harlan was the only veteran I'd met who knew much of anything about Vietnam prior to his deployment there. Upon getting his orders, he went to his local library to do research; he wanted to discover where he was being sent and the reason he was going to war.

That wasn't supposed to matter to a Marine infantryman. But it did to him. If he was going to kill the enemy, he wanted to know exactly who he was killing and why.

When he arrived in Vietnam, it didn't take long before he learned for himself why he *wasn't* fighting. It wasn't the reasons in the headlines. As his tour wore on, Harlan's cynicism chiseled away the war's lies. Under that pile of rubble was the naked truth:

Their lives didn't matter.

He and his fellow Marines were only special to those that loved them. To the politicians who sent them to war, their lives were not precious. They were expendable.

And in Harlan's judgment, they gave their lives for no good reason. They were not there to win the war. They were not there for God and country. Neither were they there to seize land nor seek glory in the spoils of winning. Their job was simple and very much to the point:

They were there to count bodies.

And to him, it didn't matter whose bodies they counted. The politicians just needed more of them so they could make the defense contractors rich off of the blood of America's youth.

For twelve months, he saw too much death and wondered every day when it would be his turn. He questioned how many bodies it would take for people to wake up and see the madness of the war for what it was.

He now understood why the veterans with the most time in country had that far-off look in their eyes. They saw the truth. If they couldn't escape the insanity, perhaps they could disengage their soul to numb the pain. He heard the mantra repeated over and over....

"Yeah, it don't mean nuthin.' Not a thing...."

Harlan watched as young Marines cycled in and out of I Corps, only to become another body to be counted. And so it went. Shortly after zipping their mangled remains into bags, their replacements would get off the chopper, eyes wide.

It usually took months for their thousand-yard stare to set in. He eventually stopped asking their names because it didn't matter anymore. They were simply waiting for their turn. Waiting to be counted, just like the rest of them.

As a twenty-year-old Sergeant, Harlan could no longer justify the deaths of his men, but that didn't stop the missions from coming. While his superiors assured them they were winning, he wrestled with the unconscionable price. However, as a squad leader, he couldn't free himself from the chain of command dictating their fates. One by one, they met theirs.

The smothering lies, hypocrisy, and death stoked the embers of his anger. Like the white phosphorus they used against their enemy, once it started burning, it didn't stop.

The pain came first. Then, the nightmares.

And that's when Harlan began sleeping with the dead. Though he didn't realize it then, if he made it out of this place alive, he would sleep with them the rest of his life.

Harlan wanted vengeance.

He wanted payment for his dead Marines. He wanted revenge for baking in the merciless sun, waiting for the opportunity to kill the enemy in a futile effort to make the pain go away. He wanted payback against the faceless figures who sent his men here to die horrible deaths as they waited to be counted. He wanted....

No. Needed.

He would never get the real culprits in his gunsight. He had to settle for making his enemy pay. Pay bad.

It wasn't enough to see them die. Harlan wanted to see the life dim from the eyes of his enemy who brought him to this God-forsaken country to kill him and his friends. Someone had to pay for what was happening.

He needed a mission.

It wouldn't be long. It never was.

On June 25, 1966, Operation Jay launched a large, coordinated strike against Mỹ Phú hamlet, an enemy stronghold in Thừa Thiên Province. The Marines simultaneously attacked from the north and south while a blocking force cut off any enemy attempt to escape inland.

Those details were only important to the planners. To Harlan, it was just another day for payback. He fantasized about leaving whatever rage and pain he could with the enemy bodies lying in the stinking filth of their own rice paddies.

It took some time for the rumors to materialize. He was finally called to the CP for the mission briefing.

He had been awake for two days waiting for it to launch, but early that morning, at least for a couple of hours, some sleep mercifully found him. It would have been a welcome postponement from the war, if only he didn't have to sleep with the dead again....

As Harlan slowly walks down a hill toward the cemetery in small-town America, he can see the Marine burial detail. They are in pressed dress blues. Emotionless robots in uniform. The cemetery is well manicured with beautiful flowers placed around the gravesite.

He can see that Private First Class Gary W. Thomas has many relatives and friends who loved him very much. His high school sweetheart along with the entire graduation class of 1965 is there. The choir from the church that Gary attended as a boy is singing the old gospel song, "What a friend we have in Jesus." The choir members are singing off key on this sad day.

The minister is trying to support Mrs. Thomas to keep her from falling to the ground in agony. Her body trembles with pain and grief. Gary was the youngest of her four children and the only son. She watches the burial detail remove the flag of our country before the casket is lowered into the ground. They fold the flag neatly and present it to the Captain in charge of the detail.

The officer cites the scripted words to Mrs. Thomas. Harlan knows he has said these same words far too often to the loved ones of many dead Marines. He stiffly bequeaths the flag of our country to Mrs. Thomas as a small token for her son's life.

Harlan watches as Mr. Thomas places his arms around his wife as she holds the flag to her breast just as she did with her son eighteen years ago. Mr. Thomas won't look the Captain in the eyes. He knows he would say something that would embarrass his son in his moment of glory.

Suddenly the scene changes. The cemetery is now the rice paddy that lays to the front of their night defensive position. Everything has changed to a forbidding shade of gray and is moving ominously in slow motion. Gone are the beautiful flowers and many loved ones mourning the deceased.

The burial detail has disappeared. They have been replaced by men from Harlan's unit. They are his Marines who preceded Gary Thomas in death. They have on their dirty bloodstained combat gear with the stench of decay about them. One by one, they are standing in line waiting for Harlan to apologize to them. For some insane reason he thought he could get through one more night in this living hell without sleeping with the dead.

The flare burns out and it goes dark.

As he stares out at the rice paddy, he can faintly see two people waving their arms. He stares up at the heavens and curses God for playing tricks on his mind. Just then, another pop flare lights up the night and he can see the parents of Gary Thomas, beckoning him into the paddy.

He steps from his foxhole and slowly walks towards them. As it begins to darken again, another flare ignites as he reaches the center of the paddy, and he can see Mrs. Thomas has a sinister smirk on her face. She is standing in the mud and feces holding a dirty bloodstained flag to her breast. Mr. Thomas stands next to his wife, his body covered in blood staring at Harlan with dead eyes.

In slow motion, Mrs. Thomas unfolds the soiled flag. Her husband is wiping the blood from his body with the flag and staring at him with those lifeless eyes. Harlan begs them for their forgiveness.

Gary's mother throws the flag at his face and is yelling at him. She is screaming that this dirty bloodstained rag is not a fair trade for her baby boy. She repeats over and over that it will not bring back her baby.

Harlan begs her to take him as fair trade for what she has lost. She yells that he'd never make up for what she's lost. He looks at her through the tears he's been holding back for the last year and wishes he could sleep with the dead forever.

The flare's glow starts to fade.

Mrs. Thomas is pointing at something on the ground. Harlan can see nothing but a dark, muddy hole. Another flare illuminates the night. He peers into the hole and sees PFC Thomas in the same condition as he last remembered him. His body is torn and mutilated and very dead. It starts to move. Harlan can see Gary beckon him as if to invite him to his moment of glory. There is nothing left of his face, but somehow Harlan knows he's smiling at him.

Next to Gary is a shiny metal box with some sort of inscription on the lid. Another flare lights up the night. Harlan squints and is able to now see the etched writing.

It reads "Sergeant Harlan S. Black, United States Marine Corps, Killed in Action, Republic of Vietnam, June 25, 1966."

～

Men yelling.

Harlan awakes with a start to the sounds of Marines preparing for war. Some with fearful eyes, others with vacant eyes. All are checking their equipment, shitcanning what they don't need, and loading as much ammo as they can carry.

The Marines are lining up at the CH-46 Sea Knight helicopters that will take them into battle. They bake under the merciless tropical sun as they wait their turn to board.

More yelling. The heightening pitch of revving engines and thumping rotor blades beat the thick air. The whirlwind of dust and sweat cakes their squinting faces, hiding the fear behind burning eyes.

A familiar rush of adrenaline. It is a thin line between fear and excitement, but today, it is the latter. For some reason, Harlan needs the war now more than ever. His rage demands it.

En route. The humid air whips through the aluminum hull of the chopper. Not a word said. Most look down. The pimpled-face Marine sitting next to him kisses a silver crucifix and tucks it under a sweaty olive drab tee shirt.

Harlan feels a grin of anticipation. Gotta get to war. He can feel the surge of bloodlust coursing through him as they make the approach on LZ Shrike.

Small pencil holes of light appear in the fuselage of the descending chopper. Some startle with their sudden appearance. Darting eyes scan for where the next bullets will enter.

Silent fear spreads. Will they die before having a chance to fight back?

Another surge, reflexive anger. How many times had the enemy struck only to suddenly disappear?

More pencils of light. Fraying nerves. Harlan smiles to himself—the enemy is near. He will get his chance today.

The crew chief is wildly waving them off his aircraft. Marines spring to their feet, but it is not quick enough for him. The radio just brought word that one of squadron HMM-161's choppers was shot down and is now engulfed in flames 1,000 meters to the south of the hamlet.

The crew chief pushes them onto the ramp screaming at the queued line of warriors waiting for their turn to go into battle.

"GET OFF MY BIRD! They will get a fix on us! Get the fuck off my bird NOW!"

Harlan splashes into the stagnant water of the rice paddy. The stench of hot mud and shit fills his nostrils.

The Lieutenant is yelling commands over the accelerating whirl of the helicopter, desperate to generate the lift to make their escape. More pencils of light. A door gunner is returning fire. The stream of searing brass casings sizzle as they sink into the paddy water.

Screaming orders. The oppressive rotor wash sprays the Marines with putrid water and muffles their instructions.

"Spread the hell out people! This is Charlie's backyard. One round and you're all dead! Spread the hell out! MOVE IT!"

The sweat is stinging his eyes, but Harlan sees their objective in the tree line many hundred meters in front of them. In the distance to his left flank, faint cracking and popping.

Harlan's heart races as he tightens his grip on the battle-scarred wooden stock of his M14 rifle. Other assault teams are already in the fight. It's just a matter of time until they, too, will be in the fight. Must see their eyes.

He barely completes the thought before the indescribable sound of incoming bullets break the sound barrier. Getting closer. The enemy gunners are correcting for the distance of his approaching platoon. It's too far for accurate fire. But close enough.

More screaming. Double timing to clear the coverless kill zone.

Deadly plumes of fire, smoke, mud, and water erupt 100 meters in front of them. The shock waves reach them a moment later. The distant thump of the next volley of mortars is unmistakable. More yelling. Then the whistling.

"MOVE! MOVE IT! They have a bead on us! MOVE NOW!"

The next rounds are far closer but behind them. The air is pierced by shards of shrapnel. The enemy mortar teams now have the Marines bracketed and are walking them in. The shock waves mix with fear to propel their advance.

Finally on dry ground. More explosions. Yelling. Running now. Must clear the kill zone.

Harlan is smiling as they close on the enemy position. The swirl of fear, thrill, and rage envelopes him and threatens to hijack his body and mind. He is a hardened warrior and silently coaches himself as he runs.

"Been here before … don't panic. Shoot back. Must shoot back. You are not going to die in this stinking paddy! This is where the dead sleep. Keep running. Shoot!"

Chaotic sounds of war. He hears screaming and dying as the now-zeroed mortar rounds pummel the advancing Marines.

His squad reaches their first line of cover, a paddy dike parallel to the tree line in front of them. He can see the other squads in his periphery fanning out behind the dike in preparation to assault the tree line. As the squad leader, he is now yelling the commands.

Hearts pounding. His riflemen take aim and fire. Harlan watches in merriment as he sees the enemy fall, but he cannot see their eyes like he needs to. Gotta get closer.

He yells to his men over the cracking symphony of 7.62mm rounds and the reassuring thump of his grenadier's M79.

He sees a graveyard down range and to his right. His mind knows the plan before he can consciously assemble it. The advanced team will take up firing positions in the graveyard while he and his three less experienced riflemen cover their advance.

Word travels down the line. As if the enemy senses the threat, the incoming volume of fire increases, the rounds smacking loudly into the sunbaked clay paddy dike.

On Harlan's command, the leading fireteam takes off at a sprint while the rest lay down suppressive fire. Fire and maneuver, just as they were trained.

The enemy fire drops off into an expected lull. Then another isolated burst rings out. Harlan peers over the dike just in time to see his grenadier grotesquely crumble to the ground as if cut down by an invisible sword.

Teeth clenching. He can feel the rage bubble up from his core, but it is interrupted by bone jarring explosions.

The first volley is almost on top of them. Screams of his fireteam are cut short as they are pelted with a shower of stinking mud and debris. By now, his men taking cover in the graveyard are firing at the tree line.

Time to move. Harlan shouts his orders.

As he rises to break for the graveyard, he senses he is alone. Incredulous, he turns to see his three riflemen curled in fetal positions behind the dike.

"Get up and fight, damn you! You're MARINES!"

Bullets slicing the air. More explosions. No time left.

"On my ass, NOW!"

He sprints for the graveyard as rounds kick up the dusty earth just feet behind him. He shouldn't have to look. He doesn't have time to look. They will follow me. They are Marines. *Semper Fidelis.*

Running. Heaving. Crack of bullets trying to find him.

He is their only target. He is alone.

More sounds of war. Closer now. He can hear the thumping of mortars raining hell on the other assault teams. He is firing and running.

The sounds of war go silent. He hears only his labored breathing as he closes on the first row of graves. Suddenly, all of his senses divert inward as the wind is knocked out of him.

He feels three bullets, as if traveling in slow motion, piercing his chest, shoulder and lower back. His legs give out and he feels the unforgiving earth crash into him.

Trying to find his breath. Gasping. His lungs gurgle but fill enough to get him on his feet.

He refuses to sleep with the dead. Have to see their eyes....

Harlan staggers towards the pile that used to be his grenadier. He instinctively dips to grab the M79 grenade launcher. He feels a fleeting glimpse of pleasure—more enemy will die with this weapon of his fallen heroes.

Advancing at a broken trot, he strains to stay on his feet. It is fueled only by rage as his strength drains from his wounds. He silences the closest enemy mortar team with a well-aimed 40mm grenade.

He cracks the breach to reload, but his head spins. Gotta breathe. More gurgling. Feet will no longer carry him.

Nothing left. Won't get to see their eyes.

Harlan collapses into a gravestone and reaches for it to break his fall. He props himself against its rough stone face. He can feel the life draining from him as his blood soaks into his uniform.

Is it finally his turn? To be counted. To sleep with the dead. To have his moment of glory.

Can't keep them open. He surrenders to the unbearable heaviness of his eyelids. Fading sounds of war.

Harlan senses his body being jerked up and thrown into a poncho. More yelling. The poncho bounces to the irregular rhythm of running men.

More gunfire. A sudden fall. The hard ground and pain jolts Harlan to consciousness.

The man carrying the left side of the poncho is suddenly next to him and begins to put his forehead back together just inches from Harlan's face. He recognizes the corporal as the company brown nose—the marine who always had his nose stuck up the captain's ass.

Here was a man Harlan could never bring himself to like now risking his life to carry him to safety. He gets shot in the back of the head, but Harlan doesn't have the strength to help him find the pieces of his skull. *Semper Fidelis*.

Light dimming. Sounds of war fade to silence.

More yelling. He awakes lying among hastily assembled rows of the dead and wounded with only thin strands separating their fates. The company corpsmen are tagging bodies and zipping them into black body bags.

Distant sounds of war. In his haze, he can hear the inbound choppers in the distance. The agony of the wounded is unbearable. Harlan is making promises to God he knows he won't be able to keep. The whirlwind of dusty light fades to black.

He senses vibrations. He is not sure if his eyes are open or not—he can see nothing.

A cacophony of unbearable pain slams into him—aching, burning, stabbing. Muffled thumping. No more sounds of war. A vague awareness makes its way through his agony.

This is it. This must be hell. I now have to sleep with the dead. More blackness....

Suddenly his damaged lungs gasp for air but there is little. The pain moves to the background as his body desperately searches for a breath. His suffocation infuses another burst of adrenaline.

Harlan is trying to move his arms. He is in a dark rubber cocoon that pushes back against his feeble effort. His body is frantically lurching towards dimming life.

Muffled screaming. Rapidly shifting hands are palpable through the rubberized barrier.

Harlan is suddenly blinded by a searing beam an inch from his face. Large pencil of light.

They even shoot at you in hell....

A pressured rush of cool air pours through the widening zipper. His lungs devour it all. Pupils constrict and struggle to focus.

Yelling faces. Many hands. Further unzipping the triangular opening. Pushing on him. Pulling him. Bandaging him. He doesn't feel the sting of the needle.

A warm rush courses through his body. The agony feels further away.

Another thought through the haze. If this is hell, sleeping with the dead ain't so bad.

More blackness and shades of gray mixed with a macabre mosaic of flashbulb memories. Screams and moans of the wounded. Scrub-suited figures with surgical masks. Only round eyes show through, but they are not the eyes he needed to see. He will never get that chance again.

Bright bulbs. Hands moving over his limp body. Heavy eyelids. Dimming lights. Darkness.

It is not yet Harlan's turn to sleep with the dead. It is June 25, 1966, the day of his rebirth. Night has fallen on South Vietnam once more.

⁓

The pain slams his chest and radiates into his scarred shoulder. His legs weaken as he reaches for the wooden orchard fence to break his fall.

That sonofabitch cardiologist.

He sits propped against the weathered cedar post, almost exactly as he had thirty-nine years earlier. His pursed lips gave way to a spreading grin as the irony of his end sets in. Since then, he has slept with the dead only in his dreams. Finally, he will join them.

⁓

Epilogue: The nightmare embedded in this broader story was written by my patient and freely given to me in the context of his treatment. This dream recounted the loss of one of his Marines (whom he gave the same pseudonym used in the above story), his guilt over the deaths of those under his command, and his own near-death experience on Operation Jay on June 25, 1966. After he was shot three times in the torso and presumed dead, this veteran came to consciousness inside of a body bag on the medevac chopper. He was awarded the Silver Star for his valorous actions with the 2/1st Marines that day.

Harlan died while trimming trees in his orchard many years before this book was conceived and permission could therefore not be granted by the veteran. Next of kin was contacted and consent for this story provided on his behalf. The excerpt of this veteran's nightmare, and the story surrounding his actions that day, are included in this collection to honor his valorous service, sacrifice and years of suffering with PTSD symptoms from this trauma.

13

Promises to
One-Eyed George

I had no idea how he lost his eye. But I do know how he came to occupy the passenger seat of my Saab as I buckled in the black, scruffy mutt in for my commute home from work. I'd made a promise and I'd be damned if he was going to get injured on the 30-minute drive home because I had to stop short.

George was used to being in cars. That's how he found his way to me that day.

His owner, Silas, a USMC Vietnam combat veteran and patient of mine left him in his car the day he came to see me for his regular therapy session. George went everywhere with Silas—they were inseparable. Occasionally, Silas brought him into the building, but on that day, he didn't want George to hear what he was about to tell me.

I was aware his trauma anniversary date was coming up. What I did not yet know was what Silas planned for that hot August 21 day. It was the

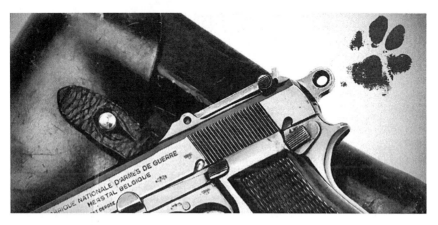

Author's photograph.

date his Marine squad in Vietnam were all killed only days after the veteran completed his thirteen-month tour and DEROS'd home. He carried the burden of survivor guilt for four decades and today, he determined he had carried it long enough.

George was actually Karl's dog. Karl served with the 101st Airborne in Vietnam, and he and Silas met in my Monday afternoon PTSD group. They became tight as their connection blossomed. However, the following year, Karl's two pack-a-day habit caught up with him. Silas, an avowed Buddhist, figured the imminent loss was his karma because of his "abandonment" of his squad. He took the news of Karl's metastatic lung cancer hard.

Karl didn't fight the news. He was tired too. But he had a couple of requests to make of his best friend. To commemorate his impending death, Silas organized the first "live wake" I ever attended. Fraternizing with patients outside of the VA environment was generally forbidden, with certain ceremonial exceptions, such as funerals. Karl wasn't dead yet, but he specifically requested my presence there. I was not going to turn down a dying man's wish.

I don't regret my decision. That was the last time I saw Karl.

Then came the second promise. As Silas swore to his dying friend, he assumed custody of George—one of his virtues was that he always kept his promises. Always.

Which is part of what scared me. In spite of years of treatment, he couldn't shake the burden of guilt for not being there to lead his squad to safety after he left Vietnam. Besides, according to Silas, if anyone deserved to live, it wasn't him. He pledged forty-five years later, to the day, he would make things right by joining his fellow squad mates in death.

"Tomorrow is the day. I just came to tell you that."

Silas both threatened and attempted suicide many times before. He was admitted to inpatient psychiatry more times than I could count. And it wasn't just the war. He was a man of many burdens and there was no telling when he might decide, as he did many times before, that he had had enough.

He lived his life in the fast lane for many years, and violence became the center of it. After Vietnam, he was recruited and served as a mercenary in the South American drug wars, later descending into the drug culture himself. At first, he served as the "muscle" in big drug deals, but later went into "business" for himself manufacturing methamphetamine in the 1980s and served three prison terms for related drug offenses.

Even when he straightened up after his last release, he lived dangerously. He was a motorcycle enthusiast, survived countless wrecks, and carried as much scar tissue as skin to prove it. Oddly, fate saved his life about as many times as he intentionally tried to end it.

I first met Silas just after he was released from his final incarceration in the mid–1990s when he presented for PTSD treatment. As he tried to step into the light for the first time since Vietnam, his past began to haunt him. He had killed many times, both in war and out. Though he was surprised it survived his sordid past, in therapy he slowly discovered that he did have a conscience; he was not, as he believed for most of his life, simply a cold-hearted killer. This only amplified his guilt.

But knowing that wasn't enough. It just wasn't about his squad. It was about a lot of things. He was in and out of treatment for many years with some progress, but not enough to end the chronic hurt. He was a haunted man, and tired of the ghosts. He wasn't in my office that day to play games. He ran out of reasons to keep going.

"So, if you want to kill yourself tomorrow, what are you doing here?"

The question was both a legitimate query and my opening move in a complex psychological chess game. He began to build his case for death. I was going to start working from the other side with the only leverage I had—beginning with faint hints of ambivalence wherever they could be found.

"I just came by to say 'thanks' and that it's not your fault. You are not responsible for this."

Silas was all too familiar with the corrosive effects of guilt—even in the myopia of his pain, he was thoughtfully trying to spare me from what was coming. And it was not an empty threat.

I knew he had a pistol; Silas purchased the 1941 Nazi-proofed 9mm Belgian Hi-Power pistol from a World War II veteran friend of his who brought it back from the campaign in Europe as a war souvenir. As a three-time felon, he wasn't supposed to have it, but the law never was much of an obstacle for Silas.

As I weighed the situation, the risk factors continued to pile up; his depression worsened as August approached, and his trauma anniversary date was tomorrow. His endless struggle to function was continuing unabated in spite of many intervention efforts. He also had a history of impulsive decision making, and he was ready to end the pain. I knew him too well to risk playing the odds.

As we talked, I could see him slowly making his way towards reconsideration, but he wasn't making it easy. He was smart enough to see through my line of inquiry and the logic on which I was building my case. He countered every question and I was running low on ideas. As the dialogue continued, I maneuvered towards the one question that appealed to his virtues and that I was hoping would tip the balance in favor of life.

"And what about George?"

I saw his face register a direct hit.

Aside from always keeping his promises, the other thing that I knew about Silas was that he was an animal lover. A dog lover to be exact. I believed he didn't mind killing himself, but leaving George homeless was an entirely different matter. Intense loyalty and keeping his word weren't just a thing with him—they were everything to him.

After the living wake, Silas' second promise was to care for George. If he didn't want me to find that pressure point, then he shouldn't have told me many months earlier that he made that exact pledge just before Karl's death.

"Oh yeah … shit…. George…. He's in the car."

The conversation went on from there. We both sensed without saying it that he just needed a face-saving way out. With my help, he was also glimpsing the irony of violating his promise to Karl, compromising his word, and doing so to commemorate his loyalty and grief over his best friends who were killed in Vietnam.

Before he changed his mind, he made one last weary thrust. "I'm just tired of living with the pain of letting my friends down. They died while I saved my own skin and left that damn place. And this is about the only way I know to make it right."

I carefully took aim at the most obvious weak link.

"I am trying to understand how breaking your word to Karl, abandoning George, and taking your own life is honoring your dead friends. You couldn't save your friends then and you cannot save them now. But you can consider using your pain to do something good with it by taking care of George. He needs you. That might be the way you make things right."

I paused a moment for impact.

"Besides … you promised."

That did it. I could see the shift in him as he contemplated the possibility of allowing all of that to be true.

Silas didn't have a lot of formal education, but he was smart. Even in the cloud of his moral anguish, the dissonance expanded and his reasoning collapsed. I could see the muscles shift in his jaw and then relax as he surrendered.

He tensed for a moment and looked at the floor as I watched him continue to search for an honorable way to break his plan to end his life. That was my cue and I opened the door for him.

"How about you just come into the hospital for a little bit until we get through your trauma anniversary?"

We agreed that he needed an admission to ensure he'd survive the day, but we had a problem.

"What about George? I can't be admitted. He's in the car. How about if I find someone to watch him and I come back tomorrow?"

I immediately vetoed that idea. There was that other time he left our session and bought a bottle of vodka on the way home with the intent to get drunk before shooting himself. Had he not passed out and a friend dropped by to see him asleep on the couch with that 9mm pistol on his table, I might never have learned of that close call. That was only a couple of years ago.

After he was admitted to the hospital, he spilled what triggered that attempt.

For months, Silas eyed a vintage pocket watch at a local pawn shop. But he couldn't bring himself to buy it. It was too expensive, he told himself. We later uncovered the deeper truth in a subsequent therapy session: he couldn't offer a gift of such opulence to himself, and worse, didn't feel worthwhile enough to deserve such a fine watch.

It took several months to chisel through that belief. Fatefully, the watch waited until he believed he mattered enough to own it.

One day, he came to session beaming. He purchased the watch on his way to our appointment. His intent was to show it to me in a major symbolic and emotional victory for him. However, that day, he forgot two things.

He forgot the watch which lay on the passenger seat.

And he forgot to lock the car's doors.

"I can't believe I forgot it. I'll show you next time," Silas offered, a bit embarrassed by his absent-mindedness.

Only there wouldn't be a next time. He parked by the outdoor smoking shelter in front of the substance abuse treatment building. The shelter was loaded with veterans, some of whom were trying to get clean and go straight, and some who hadn't given up their old ways.

Silas walked out of session beaming with a nascent pride only to discover the evidence of what he assumed was the bitter truth; he shouldn't have owned that watch anyway. Fate confirmed it—he didn't deserve anything good.

On the way home that day, he drove to the liquor store. He lived alone, so he had time. Time to get numb once more. Time before pulling the trigger. It would be the final pull in a life filled with too many of them. After his knocking went unanswered, his neighbor let himself in only to find Silas in a stupor, with that loaded Nazi pistol on the coffee table.

No—while we made substantial progress since that last close call, I didn't trust that he wouldn't change his mind between now and tomorrow.

"I really believe you need to come in right now."

But we had a problem. That problem was sitting in the car eagerly awaiting Silas' return.

The negotiations continued as we went down the checklist of possible surrogate caretakers for George. Unfortunately, Silas's limited social support system was unreliable and he wasn't going to be admitted only to abandon George to chance.

He wouldn't have dared suggested it, but I figured it was the only way.

"I'll take him," I heard myself say.

"You would do that for *me*?"

"Sure." We both smiled at the mental handshake which probably saved his life.

The only remaining problem was that no one had included George in this decision.

As I buckled the seatbelt across his shaggy body, he seemed compliant enough. No problem, I told myself. Since he was used to waiting in cars, I stopped on the way home and bought a couple of cans of gourmet dog food. If George was going to be my guest, he was going to eat well.

Upon our arrival, my two-grade school-aged children erupted.

"Daddy got us a dog!!"

With deflated faces, they digested the disappointing truth. The kids settled for playing fetch and marveled that a dog with one eye didn't have any problems catching and returning a tossed tennis ball. George was friendly enough, quite adaptable, and seemed surprisingly comfortable with his new playmates in his temporary home.

That is, until it was time for bed.

Silas didn't offer many instructions, so I was unaware that George was not used to sleeping alone. Silas shared that when he would have nightmares of Vietnam, George was always there to lick his face, and ground him when he woke up, disoriented, covered in sweat, and in a panic.

I, on the other hand, was not used to sleeping with a dog.

So, as we approached bedtime, my plan was to barricade George in the kitchen for the night. The kids thoroughly enjoyed making a bed for him out of pillows and blankets, and after an extended session of assuring affection to settle him in, I turned off the light, said goodnight to George, and started up the stairs.

That was not George's plan. It started as a lonely "woof," though after going unanswered, George stepped up his protest.

By the time I came back down the stairs, he had easily cleared the make-shift barricade and was in the living room wagging his tail furiously and crouching, rump in the air, in joyful defiance.

I might have been able to talk someone out of killing themselves, but George was not going to be persuaded to spend the night alone. He missed Silas and quickly taught me that I was no match for his will. I tried several more times to put him back in the kitchen to show him who was in charge.

He would have none of it. He would bark even louder, and like Pavlov's dogs in reverse, I quickly responded by trying to quiet him with reflexive petting and more affection. The barking stopped instantly. George's human conditioning experiment was a smashing success and lasted until the early hours of the morning.

George and I ended up eventually "sleeping" in the basement together. When the alarm sounded, I thought surely this must have been a cruel mistake. But George was ready. He seemed rather smitten with himself as we drove back to the VA, belted into my passenger seat, perfectly behaved, as if it were his daily commute.

I unbelted and leashed George before heading towards the trauma recovery unit. I could hear her the second I entered the floor; my nurse manager threw her head back, her familiar cackle greeting us as we continued wearily up the hall. I had called ahead on the way to work, told her of our adventure last night and, out of pity, she agreed to take George off my hands for the following night.

This became a team effort and we all learned important lessons about loyalty, relationships and, above all, the importance of trust and keeping one's word. Silas was alive and safe in the hospital, George was not abandoned, and the binding promises of all of us to take care of the black one-eyed dog were kept.

~

Epilogue: Silas survived ten more years. He stayed in therapy, took his medication, and though he continued to suffer from severe bouts of depression and chronic suicidal impulses, he never again attempted to kill himself following this hospitalization. He continued to work through his moral pain in treatment. And he kept his pact with Karl and provided George with a loving home until the dog peacefully passed away.

He would go on to adopt another rescue cat and eventually another rescue dog until his own death a few years later. Though Silas did not die by his own hand, he eventually found the peace that proved so elusive to him in life. However, he died knowing that he kept his promise to his friends—all of them.

14

Lost in the Woods

Though I'd never seen it before, I knew exactly what it was the instant his widow pulled it out of her purse and laid it upon my desk. The emotional connection with Wes that channeled through its presence in my office was overpowering.

My eyes locked onto the compass with the homemade braided lanyard on my desk. It was graced with a fine patina to match its age. His father passed it down to Wes just prior to his death. Now in my own grief, my mind connected it to the man I worked with for many years and who was now dead by his own hand.

Coming home from the war was rough on Wes. After serving in a combat psychological operations unit in Vietnam, he searched for ways to reintegrate back into his rural Illinois home. However, his experience of "home" just wasn't the same upon his return. He changed profoundly during the war and would never be the same.

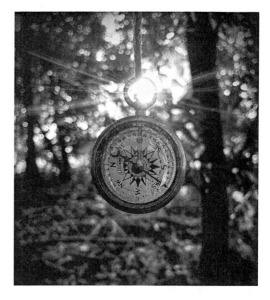

But Wes eventually settled down, had a family, and went to work as a heavy equipment operator for the state highway department. He was also an avid hunter and consummate woodsman. As his son came of age, Wes became involved in scouting, a perfect match for his expertise in survival skills and love of

Author's photograph.

the outdoors. He was so at home in the forest that he referred to it as his church—the church of "father son and mother earth." Because they embodied his spirituality, those same words were later inscribed on his tombstone.

As was typical for the years that Wes saw me for his war traumas, he came into therapy jumpy, restless, and with a slight tremor reflecting his near constant overactive arousal. Though he eventually came to trust me, he didn't even feel safe in my office. I soon learned this wasn't personal. My guest chairs would have put his back to the door; he couldn't tolerate that. He always moved his seat off to the side so he could watch the door out of the corner of his eye while we talked. The only place Wes truly felt at peace was in the woods.

Well … most of the time.

One day he called me in a panic after returning from a morning of deer hunting. He experienced a flashback and he was reeling from his reliving of an overwhelming combat incident we had not yet discussed. By the time I was able to piece together what happened during the hunt, Wes was gradually gaining his composure as the picture finally emerged to explain his surreal experience that day.

He shot at and missed a deer. This wasn't an unusual circumstance for a deer hunter except for one reason: Wes didn't miss while hunting—ever. This crisis in the woods opened the portal, and he finally told me the story behind the trigger for his flashback.

I came to learn that he did miss a shot....

Once.

It was during the war and the historic rhyme to his hunt. It was also the reason his traumatic past suddenly invaded his consciousness while in his deer stand that crisp November morning. In Vietnam, Wes missed the most important shot of his life and that is why he couldn't forgive himself—it hurt too bad.

It was not his marksmanship. He missed because he was stuck between a morally impossible choice he could never reconcile. As a result, the shot he missed on that mission in 1968 haunted him ever since.

On one side of that choice was his best friend and squad mate, Pete. He took a concealed position on Wes's flank about seventy-five meters away in full view of the village they were monitoring for enemy activity that hazy morning.

On the other side of that choice was a child. From his position, Wes watched incredulously as a woman from the village directed a young Vietnamese boy carrying a satchel charge towards his best friend's observation point. From his vantage, Pete couldn't see the child; he was unaware of the approaching danger until it was too late.

His mind raced. Wes had to act. He desperately tried to warn him, but was unable to attract Pete's attention. He tried hand signals to no avail and then relied on the intuitive ability to communicate with one another's mind they developed over time from their combat-borne symbiotic bond.

But the message never reached him.

In recounting that mission in session, Wes swore that the telepathic connection they shared was broken the night before during a rare dispute. Pete made a grievous mistake, and though he begged for Wes's forgiveness, the rupture required more time to resolve.

Time they didn't have. The mission the following day wouldn't afford it.

Without any ability to warn Pete, Wes watched in helpless horror as the window of critical decision-making quickly closed with each of the boy's hurried steps.

Wes was raised on a farm. His father taught all of his children to shoot and hunt from a very young age. Their ability to feed their large family counted on that skill and they all took that training very seriously. Wes always remembered his father's stern instruction around firearm safety:

"Don't you ever point your weapon at another person…. EVER…."

Wes struggled with this injunction after he arrived in Vietnam. But it dimmed soon after he killed his first man and all but disappeared after months in the bush. But this was different. This was a child.

He heard his father's words as his mind raced to search for a solution to stop what he saw coming. He reflexively raised his M16 rifle, took aim, and fired.

Though what happened next was a blur in his memory, Wes could only recount the deafening detonation and the blinding flash of light.

When the shock began to subside, yells of villagers sounding the intruder alarm jolted him. His position was compromised, and he had to get out quickly. To his great shame, the most potent piece of the memory was his panicked exfiltration and three smothering moral realizations: that Pete and the child were both dead … he had no choice but to leave his friend behind….

…and that he missed.

We tried to fill in the gaps of his account in therapy, but it was fuzzy. He swore he missed the shot, and, in the final analysis, his recollections were all we had.

We looked at the mission from every conceivable angle, slowly turning the situation from one painful facet to the next. We started with his base premise—his sworn testimony that he tried to stop the child but missed his shot.

Perhaps he hit the satchel charge and detonated it. If that were true, he concluded he would have been responsible for killing both Pete and the boy. If he cleanly missed his target, the boy would have closed the distance and detonated the explosion which ultimately killed them both. If his shot had hit its mark, he would have slain a child. Did his shock of being faced with the impossible cause him to hesitate too long?

For Wes, there was no way out—it was a psychological Gordian knot that neither of us could undo. Missing the shot the opening morning of deer season turned out to be the conduit through which the horrifying past and the unbearable present melded together, and forced him to relive those moments of fear and anguish.

After his deer season, we continued to wrestle with that knot. The best we could do was to honor the impossible choice he was forced to make and the stark dilemma of what was right, and what was necessary. Often in trauma therapy, embracing our human limitations in the face of the impossible offers the only way out. It is not an answer that comes easy to most warriors.

As we contemplated this revelation, Wes abruptly changed the subject.

He wanted to tell me about how he once helped another person who was lost. Normally, I would redirect his avoidance back to the wound. I didn't this time. I just listened.

The story was allegorical and important for us both to hear in that moment. It was about the patinaed compass that, years later, his widow pulled out of her purse and laid upon my desk.

⁓

It was the dawn of another hot and humid midwestern summer day. The boy scout troop worked its way through the hardwood forest on an early morning orientation exercise.

Wes was the last pack leader in the loose string of scouts learning to master the use of a compass to navigate through the woods. The column stretched thinner as the boys were separated in the thick green underbrush and the older scouts steadily advanced further ahead.

Though Wes loved the woods, on this particular day, its sensory details were just too close. The heat. The thick air. The buzzing insects. The potent sun filtering through the layers of foliage to the forest floor. Green everywhere.

His ears perked. His eyes darted back and forth as the collective voices of the forest created ghosts in his mind. At every step, he carefully planted the heel of his hiking boot before silently rolling it into the soft earth. He caught himself looking and listening for those who might be lying in ambush. Like that day in the woods, sometimes the combination rhymed too much, and he sensed the jungle drifting back into him. The sniffling sounds of a boy in distress snapped him into the present.

Wes found a young scout leaning against a tree. He was crying and holding his compass in his hand. By then, the voices of his scout pack faded as the rest of the column advanced beyond view.

"What's wrong?"

"I don't understand how to use this," the boy shamefully admitted while holding out his compass. "I was just following them. Now I'm lost." His eyes filled again.

Wes squatted down level with the boy's flushed face.

"Do you want me to teach you how to use that? That way, you'll never have to follow anyone ever again."

The boy stopped crying and studied Wes's face, soaking in his sincerity.

Wes took the patinaed compass with the homemade lanyard from around his neck. It was the same compass his father used to teach him. The boy raised his own compass to follow along in the instruction.

He showed his student how to find the northern heading and follow an azimuth. He explained how this established his direction towards the waypoints that would help him find his way out of the forest.

The boy mimicked his instructor, found his heading and followed its guidance through the trees, slowly looking back for assurances. Wes smiled and nodded, and the boy's pace began to steady, then accelerate.

He didn't look back again.

Wes and I sat together for a moment in silence letting the healing tale sink in. We began to discuss what it meant to him.

He helped a scared boy find his confidence and rescue himself from lostness. He helped another find his way out of the woods that he both loved but was often lost in himself, especially when the forest and jungle became one. In spite of his demons, helping others became Wes' new mission; he was always the first one to drop everything to help another, but searched his entire adult life to learn how to help himself find his way out.

A way out of those woods.

I can't honestly say Wes ever found the hoped-for-relief from this moral injury about the day Pete died. How I wish we could have found the healing he needed and deserved.

And that is why I cherished and remembered the story of the compass. Not simply because it offered some comfort while we wrestled in therapy with the pain of a dark chapter in Wes's life; it was a redemptive, hopeful trope in its own right: it was a story of coming-of-age, a father-figure passing down his wisdom to a child, and most importantly, helping one who was lost find his way.

But it was also about us. Together, we journeyed that wooded path to find our way out of his own emotional lostness. Perhaps for those reasons, Wes needed to tell the story on that day. And I needed to hear it.

Wes never found his way out of those woods. Many years later, for reasons I still cannot fully comprehend, he took his own life. The context of the period leading to that day was immensely complicated, but all efforts to save him were, ultimately and painfully, to no avail. I will never know exactly what role that impossible choice, those he couldn't save, and the unsolvable angst played in his death. I only know that Wes came back from Vietnam profoundly wounded, and that he never recovered from the day Pete and that boy died.

But I knew one thing about Wes and his story of the compass—the day he found the lost boy in the forest, I was certain he saved one.

II

Transformation
and Return

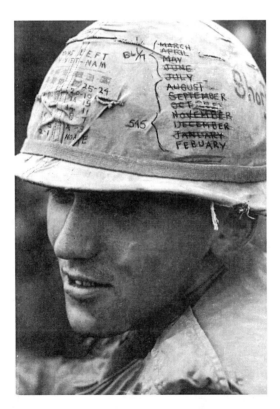

1st Cavalry Sky Trooper with short-timers helmet cover. National Archives.

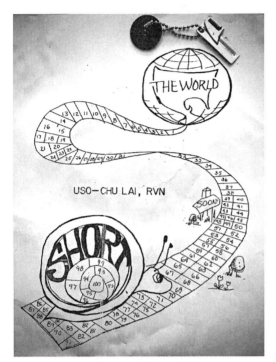

Short timer's calendar and P38 can opener.

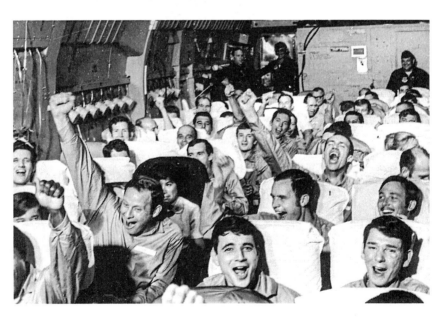

Former American POWs cheering as they take off from Hanoi, Vietnam, during Operation Homecoming, 1973. National Archives.

15

Silent Night

The gentle glow of candle flames filtered through the parting elevator doors. Marvin's pupils constricted in response to the rows of tea lights framing both sides of the dim main floor corridor of San Francisco's David Grant Medical Center at Travis Air Force Base.

Dressed in their holiday best, the civilian choral group beamed in unison with the appearance of the newly arrived men of honor they awaited. The six new patients, exhausted from their medical transport from Japan just two nights ahead of Christmas, wearily exited the elevator.

The leader signaled the carolers with a lone, angelic G note. The corridor filled with the soul-stirring harmony that the returning wounded warriors last heard a lifetime ago. Struck motionless by nostalgia, they stood in the haunting embrace of now-alien feelings that disappeared somewhere in the jungle.

"Silent Night, Holy Night.... All is calm, all is bright...."

It just didn't fit anymore. The fresh ivory bandages that encircled their bodies couldn't hold back that truth.

Tears streamed down Marvin's stubbled cheeks.

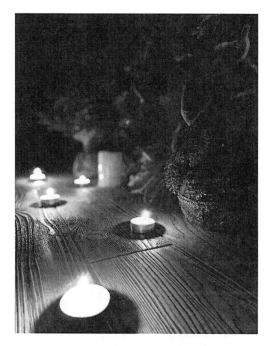

Author's photograph.

127

⌒

Ronnie was in country less than a month before a short American mortar round ended his short life. The military shrouded the painful truth that he was accidentally killed with their own ordnance during an enemy engagement with its unapologetic euphemisms; his cause of death was categorized, as were other casualties of friendly fire, as "misadventure."

Ronnie was twenty years old, and the only friend in Vietnam Marvin could count from his hometown. They attended the same high school, played on the football team, and were members of the 4-H tractor club. When they discovered themselves serving together in the 9th Infantry Division in the Mê Kông Delta, the bond was instantaneous—and in their new horror, the sole comfort of the familiar.

It was October 13, 1968. That day, Ronnie's body was laid to rest in Grimes-Neeley Cemetery in Jerseyville, Illinois. Eight thousand miles away, the descending formation of Hueys flared as they closed to a hover into the hot LZ. Muzzle flashes flickered in the deep shadows of the tree line. Incoming rounds snapped the tropical air as Marvin's infantry squad jumped from the skids and scrambled for cover under the deafening rhythm of the door gunners' suppressive M60 fire.

For Marvin, after Ronnie died, nothing was the same. But the war didn't care. It enveloped them and, bit by bit, silently began replacing the person they were with the one they were becoming. Its stealth was undetectable; its presence announced itself only when the once-familiar no longer brought comfort, leaving its emptied host with the jolting realization of the theft.

Somewhere along the way, their eyes reflected what was stolen from them. It left behind only a vacant stare—one which looked right through a person at some distant focal point a thousand yards away. Before it was all over, with bodies or souls, the war filled the butcher's bill, one way or another.

But it didn't keep those in charge from trying to hold the illusion together; the field kitchens were hard at work creating another one.

Marvin led his muddy squad in from the field to the base camp at Rạch Kiến greeted by aromas that were not of this place. They belonged to the same distant world he once inhabited during what seemed like another lifetime ago. By now, it was just another day at war, and the date just didn't matter anymore. Unless a man was "short," a calendar had no place in the field.

But the unmistakable aromas of roasting turkey and its cornucopia of fixings beckoned Marvin back to a more civilized time—it could only be the final Thursday of November.

The mess tent looked the same as always, if not noticeably busier and messier. The clanging of ladles on cavernous aluminum cauldrons radiated from the belly of the kitchen. Clouds of steam rolled through the pitched canvas ceiling before escaping from its edges only to evaporate in the blast furnace of the relentless afternoon sun. Sweating profusely, cooks and those unlucky enough for KP duty scurried about though the stifling heat and impossibly thick air. Stacked in hastily assembled rows, the insulated mermite containers patiently sat at the foot of the serving tables, preserving the warmth of the chow line's feast while the cooks furiously worked on additional batches.

Marvin's weary troops dropped their gear while their growling stomachs followed the wafting promise of something special. Each picked up a metal tray at the head of the long table and began filling its stamped sections with the Army's version of Thanksgiving Day fare.

Marvin numbly filled his tray with what would easily be his best meal since landing in Vietnam. He could hear the others pilling their trays high as the excited banter at the chow line reflected the anticipation of their first real turkey dinner. Up to that point, the only meal masquerading as such was the congealed salty turkey loaf C-ration B3A unit that came from the World War II-era olive drab cans.

After topping all but the sliced rounds of canned cranberry sauce with a ladle of thick steaming gravy, Marvin took his place at a table and prepared to dig in. He shoveled a bite into his mouth.

The tastes were all there, but something was wrong. He tried another bite, but the feeling wouldn't leave—it only became stronger. The nagging visceral sense then attached to the memory that explained it.

Marvin went back to the last Thanksgiving meal he could remember. He grew up on a farm in rural Southern Illinois. While his family holidays were not exactly the Norman Rockwell ideal, the felt sense and concept of giving thanks for the bounty of the earth was clear and unmistakable. Back in the world, Thanksgiving Day meant something.

He sat at the table lost in reflection trying to gather the over-chewed mouthful to get it down, but his throat fought back. His body led; his mind followed. Another thought entered a moment later—then a flood of them all at once.

He continued turning the puzzle piece of what Thanksgiving meant to him every which way, trying to jam it into the unwilling world in which he now lived. He thought about what he was doing with a rifle in a country so far from home on this hallowed day. He thought about what he was fighting for and why. All the while, he kept rotating the puzzle piece of the now-incongruous holiday, slowly at first, then frantically, looking for a way to make it fit the jagged edges of the war.

In the middle of straining to swallow a third mouthful, Marvin got up from the table, and dumped a meal that many in the field would have killed for into the empty garbage can.

Five days later, it was just another dateless day.

Another day of war.

Another day on patrol.

Another day hunting the enemy.

Another day staying alive.

Marvin's patrol cautiously passed by an old, abandoned French farmhouse. The inhospitable climate of the Vietnamese jungle gradually ate into the decaying stucco as if trying to erase this crumbling vestige of French colonialism. The squad cleared the uninhabited structure and continued down the path to their objective. Viet Cong activity in this AO was steadily increasing. American patrol activity followed closely behind. Marvin's point man, Alabama, signaled and the squad silently stopped and got low.

There was nothing mysterious about his nickname. He just happened to have been from that state and with his unmistakable, thick southern drawl, he just fit his new name too well. The jungle further honed his rural senses to a fine edge and he was good on point. Marvin sent Alabama to recon the suspicious area ahead, before following him down the trail to cover his back.

The carefully camouflaged gate blended almost perfectly into the surrounding jungle. After determining it needed to be blown, Alabama started back to the squad to report his discovery. Marvin read his body language and also turned; however, his feet weren't rotating with the rest of his body. He looked at the ground to discover his jungle boots ensnared in a serpentine tangle of vines.

In Vietnam, a man could not afford even the slightest degree of inattention from the immediate. A distraction, however brief, could cost your life or that of others. But sometimes, in a moment of cosmic intervention, it may prevent you from losing the only life you had to give.

To this day, Marvin can remember little more of that moment other than the approaching cloud of dust and the concussion that slammed into his body. He recalled as he looked at his entangled feet into order to free them, his right bicep exploded in a spray of blood.

As he lay in the jungle, the darkness of unconsciousness began to lift. His senses came back in an uneven mosaic. He wasn't sure if he was dead or alive. He recalled thinking they walked into an ambush. He assumed he was knocked down by the explosion of the opening RPG that triggered the attack.

But there was nothing: no gunfire, no explosions, no yelling ... only silence.

There was no ambush—just a lone chi-com grenade whose tripwire was so well hidden that it evaded even the sharpened skills of the point man from Alabama. The booby-trapped grenade protected the gate which, they would later find out, guarded the largest VC equipment and provisions cache discovered to date in their Delta area of operations.

Marvin learned the epilogue of his patrol's story while undergoing reconstructive surgeries at Fitzsimons hospital in Denver months after being evacuated. There he ran into another soldier from his platoon on convalescent leave after being wounded during battle on January 25, 1969. In the course of those updates, Marvin heard the grim news that Jimmy Luckey, the medic who tended to his own grenade wounds that day on the patrol, and his platoon leader, Roger Vickers, were killed in that same battle.

As the squad radioed for help and began administering first aid to their two wounded men, Marvin's fuzzy sensorium trickled back. He could feel the burning pain waking to his scattered pattern of shrapnel wounds. The right side of his body had taken the brunt of the blast. It could have been worse.

He laid there while Jimmy Luckey worked on him, as another man from his squad presented Marvin with his helmet. The front of the sun-bleached olive drab cloth cover was shredded by the grenade's shrapnel. Later, he would have time to appreciate the serendipitous distraction of the tangle of vines under his feet; had he not been looking down at them when the grenade exploded, his face would have looked like his helmet.

Through the confusion and pain, Marvin dimly heard Alabama yelling about "a fuckin' tripwire." Though closer to the grenade, he was on the wayward side of a tree because of his path of return.

The VC knew what they were doing. Had Alabama tripped the wire while approaching the gate, he would have been KIA. It was by happenstance that upon his return to the squad, his lead boot caught the wire. While the life-saving tree sheltered the rest of his body from the blast, some shrapnel embedded in his right thigh and buttock.

While Marvin felt the pressure of bandages circling his limbs, the morphine brought a spreading wave of relief. The pain was still there, but further away. The flurry of activity of being medevac'd from the field receded from consciousness as the opiate slowly found each of the scattershot holes in his body and mercilessly quieted their screams.

~

Marvin awoke lying on an operating table at the 3rd Surgical Hospital in Đồng Tâm. After triage, a nurse taped off his IVs and prepped him for surgery. She assured that he was next in queue after the surgeon was done with the only other patient in the operating room. She opened the curtain cordoning off the room's sections and disappeared.

Marvin heard an unmistakable commotion and turned his head.

His eyes darted around the chaotic scene. On the OR table across the room lay the patient ahead of him. Even through his dulled pain, Marvin felt the growing burn of anger course throughout his body.

Blood was everywhere. The grievously wounded patient had hardly an uninjured part of his body exposed. All four limbs had inflatable splints while blood-soaked dressings futilely held his grotesquely mangled body together.

A visibly rattled surgeon was working on this hopeless patient while two men with intelligence insignias toggled between interrogating this dying man and prodding the doctor to do whatever it took to keep him alive. During this process, Marvin overheard the heated exchange between the doctor and the interrogators over their "methods."

It was a protest that the frustrated surgeon lost. He was quickly reminded that it may have been his OR, but he was not the one in charge.

Marvin couldn't believe what he was seeing, nor could he quell his anger. The man responsible for his delayed care was his enemy.

The battalion surgeon struggled with that very same feeling for different reasons. He was being forced to prolong his doomed patient's suffering. That he was Viet Cong didn't matter—his sworn Hippocratic oath, "Above all do no harm," was not calling the shots.

In spite of his agony, the wounded combatant twisted and writhed to evade his relentless interrogators. Marvin's anger began to fade as he watched this act of determined resistance.

Somewhere in those moments, rather than seeing his enemy, he saw a soldier who, against all hope, was conducting himself as he had wished he would if the situation were reversed. He watched the man's vigor fade as the fight in him slowly drained out of the countless holes in his body.

With a final death rattle, the contortion of his facial muscles melted into calm stillness while his pupils dilated until they settled in a final frozen gaze. The intermittent beep tracking the patient's weakening pulse gave way to an unbroken whine. The interrogators flagellated the doctor, who was now beyond their threats. He propped up his stained, gowned body on his former patient's operating table, shaking his head, and staring straight down at the spreading crimson pool on the floor in which he now stood.

The two men at the head of the table looked at each other with expressionless faces. A curt nod was exchanged between them before walking out of the doctor's OR without so much as a word, satisfied that they did everything they could to learn something—anything, that might save American lives. It was their sole mission and all that mattered anymore. Absent was any appreciation of what they lost along the way, having long-since surrendered the steep price to what was necessary.

As they prepared to leave, one of them caught an astonished stare from across the room. Marvin reflexively looked back up at the ceiling as if the interrogator's penetrating eyes might unmask his confusing emotional odyssey.

It started with anger, morphed into curiosity, and ended in respect. Harder were the feelings and thoughts that bombarded him as he made his way there. Messages that came from everywhere tried to poach him along the way. He wondered if his courage and loyalty would match that of his wounded enemy. He wrestled with the charge that respecting his enemy was offering solace, perhaps even traitorous. The interrogator's brief stare only intensified his shame.

Moments later, Marvin heard voices through masked faces offer a terse pre-op briefing. After this initial operation, he would go to Japan for additional surgeries before being flown stateside to Travis AFB in San Francisco. If all went well, he would be home by Christmas.

The pain was coming back. He just wanted to get it over with. Marvin felt a radiating coolness enter his arm and sensed the gurney beginning to roll as he slipped into unconsciousness.

It was finally his turn.

⁓

Epilogue: This was Marvin's experience of return as a medical evacuee after being wounded by a booby trap in December of 1968. Like many combat veterans, when he came home from Vietnam, nothing was the same. This story speaks to the profound changes and disconnections many experienced, including loss of relationship to friends, family, holidays, institutions, values and other foundational pillars that defined their pre-war lives.

After the military rushed him back to the United States on December 14 so he could be home by Christmas, Marvin arrived at his hometown airport to discover that no one from his family was there to greet him or welcome him home. After a solemn, lonely Christmas, Marvin reported to Fitzsimmons Army Medical Center in Denver where he spent months undergoing additional reconstructive surgeries and a long painful recovery from his war injuries.

16

Thresholds

Nico tried to adjust to the strange sensation of standing alone in his childhood home. Ever since their mom had died, his younger brother, Angelo, lived there. While he didn't keep the place up very well, he had no other place to go.

Some work injuries, and many years of living hard and fast, rendered what was left of him unable to hold down a job. Much of Angelo's spare cash went towards staying numb, and the bail bondsman took the rest. He ran with the same mafia gangster-types their father did. Too many wrong

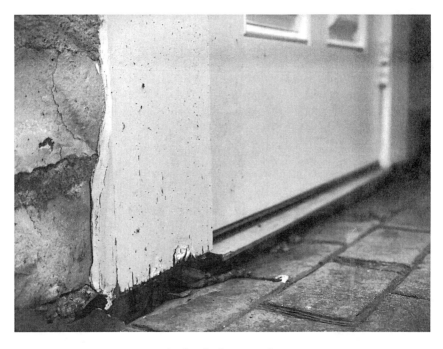

Author's photograph.

decisions put the final nails in the coffin of his independence. Now it was all up to Nico.

Considering the circumstances, the solution was a good one. To keep their parent's home in the family, Nico fixed it up and offered to cover some of the ongoing expenses so his brother could keep a roof over his head.

Whether or not Angelo's bad choices would put him out on the streets wasn't the point. No member of Nico's family would ever go unprotected—not on his watch. He knew all too well about fending for himself and covering his own back. And he paid a dear price for learning how.

At 6'4", his father bore a heavy, towering frame. His powerful hands looked like catcher's mitts. He was also a "made" man in the local mob. But it was his deep rage and hard heart that made him most dangerous.

As the eldest, Nico bore the brunt of those large, violent hands. By age fifteen, he had enough. He found his ticket out some months later when he accepted a roofing job, moved out of his family home to live with friends, and still managed to go to school when he wasn't working. In the ides of his eighteenth year, Nico escaped his father's wrath for good when he was drafted into the custody of the United States Army.

After enduring the ordeal of his childhood, getting orders for Vietnam didn't shake him. By the time Nico finished his second combat tour, he knew he could survive anything. But at this point, it was his brother he was most worried about.

Though his brother's health had been in gradual decline, Angelo's death still came as a surprise. Because Angelo was broke, he died in a stark closet-sized nook at his area hospital. Nico stood vigil by his brother's side until his very last breath. He could feel the grief tugging at him, though he had a lot of practice making such inconvenient things go away.

Besides, he had work to do.

His brother died just as he had lived. Angelo was too busy making a mess of his life to clean up after himself. While the now-eerily quiet ranch home didn't look too bad at first glance, Nico knew the basement hadn't been touched for years.

The incandescent glow of the single bulb shone upon the dim corners of his past, now blanketed in a thick layer of dusty neglect. The basement stairs creaked softly as he descended to confront it. The clock of his life turned back with each step.

Nico strained as his pupils adjusted to survey the chaotic museum testifying to his family's faded history. His father had been dead for years, but there were signs of him everywhere. As he paused on the final stair, Nico could sense an unintelligible mix of emotions stirring in his gut. He swallowed hard to keep them there. This was not going to be easy.

Silky cobwebs silently rippled in response to his entry into the stale space. A faint must of old stone and mildew greeted him. There were boxes stacked everywhere, some with a word or two hinting at their contents, others anonymous. In the far corner, sheets draped loosely over the once-familiar outlines of the old family living room set.

But "family" was a lie.

The couch was only for the adults and guests. Nico could remember the stinging, massive backhand to his cheek that reminded him of that rule. In death, it now sat as empty and unapproachable as it was in life.

So, it was neither for family nor for living. Nico smirked at the irony.

Across the room to his right, the monotoned grays were interrupted by a conspicuous burst of brightly colored oil paints. Nico's eye was immediately drawn into the welcoming arms of Jesus.

The iconic reproduction was a near-requirement for every Sicilian Catholic family and hung for years in the short hallway leading to the bedrooms. How many times as a child had he walked past that picture trying to reconcile the warmth radiating from that frozen image with the incongruous mistreatment by the man at the head of his own family table. Though Nico eventually found his way back to his faith, his family's hypocrisy drove him away from the church. The godlessness of the war in Vietnam only sealed his flight.

He cautiously approached the box containing the protruding rectangular picture. Though he couldn't yet see Judas, he felt the sting of the perfidy of men wash over him—a pain he knew well.

With each step, more of the disciples appeared. They were captured in various states of incredulity after the announcement of the imminent betrayal. Nico smirked again, wondering why they were so surprised.

In mid-thought, he froze as he caught a glint of metal. Though it was barely visible, he instantly recognized its form. How could he forget?

A flood of feelings, body sensations, and vivid images rushed at him. It hung in the same hallway as the last supper and was one of many adorning every space in the house. But this one was special—it was from the old country. The cross a pewter Christ hung upon was constructed of solid olive wood right out of Sicilian groves tended by generations of his ancestors.

The horrifying movie played back in his head. Nico could repeatedly feel its sharp corners ripping his shirt and stinging his back as his father maniacally struck him with the crucifix over and over.

Nico couldn't remember what he did to deserve that particular beating, but that didn't surprise him. Only occasionally could he connect an obvious mistake to the violence that befell him. He had long given up trying to decipher consequences at the hands of his father.

He could remember the day he caught the attention of Sister Ellen at his parochial school. She gasped at the red patches unevenly seeping through his white button-down shirt that morning. Even after calling his parents into school, his father wouldn't own up to what he did to his fourteen-year-old son.

Shocked by his denial, the Nun took a more direct approach. And she had leverage. After he lost his job at the railroad, the school agreed to a hardship tuition waiver until he got back on his feet. When Sister Ellen played that card, she finally got his father's attention. Money always did.

Nico never went to school again wearing evidence of his father's abuse. While the worst was behind him, the only way to make it end for good was to leave home. Winding up in Vietnam was hardly an escape, but at least there he had a weapon and a fighting chance.

After revisiting that atrocious chapter of his life, the beckoning odor of the subterranean room filled his nostrils to lead the way back. He stood motionless trying to anchor himself to the assuring, solid presence of the basement's stone floor.

While rummaging through another stack of boxes, he discovered an aging piece of masking tape with a few visible block letters. The oxidized label curled at the edges. When he saw his handwriting, his stomach started churning—even with the limited hint, his gut knew the contents before he did.

He drew a deep breath and slowly spread the scrolling ends of the tape. Though he forgot where he had put the cardboard box after sealing it fifty years ago, he could remember the day he wrote those letters in now-faded black marker.

"WAR SLIDES '68."

⌒

After escaping his father's wrath, bootcamp didn't affect Nico the way it hit the other recruits. He figured there was little the U.S. Army could do to him that hadn't already been done. While the drill instructors broke down the other men to rebuild them into soldiers, Nico excelled. His trainers saw his potential and after graduation in late 1967, he was off to Ft. Benning to join a new counterinsurgency training program.

The military was trying to adapt to the guerrilla warfare they encountered in South Vietnam. Hunting the enemy in the jungle required different tactics than the massed troop battles of past wars. They didn't pick just anyone to be part of their new, elite dog-handlers program, but Nico was christened with the rarely assigned MOS of 11F4D. Nico would serve as a forward scout-dog handler with the 1st Infantry Division.

His job was to walk point with his specially trained K9 in search of the enemy. They excelled in clearing booby traps and alerting his handler to the sights, sounds, and smells of danger that were beyond the senses of men. Life expectancy for the role, based on their young data set, was measured in months.

Nico survived not one tour, but two. Out in the bush, he seasoned quickly into an exquisitely tuned jungle fighter. By the time he re-upped for his second tour in December of 1968, he was promoted to the rank of non-commissioned officer.

There was little that shocked his sensibilities anymore, though just when he kept believing it couldn't get any worse, it somehow always did. And the worse it got, the dimmer the light in his soul became. It had to in order to protect him from the evil surrounding him.

~

The row of bound enemy prisoners squatted before them. Nico was attached to a LRRP team when they caught movement on the trail they were surveilling. They were hunting for human intel, not body count. And that day, they scored a prize catch.

One of the five enemy soldiers they caught was an NVA paymaster. In his satchel was a treasure trove of maps and actionable intelligence written in both Vietnamese and Russian. This was no small find. The team captured them, but that's where their roles ended.

A CIA field officer accompanied their patrol for just such a lucky occasion. This agency man was the one conducting the interrogations. He drew his .45 Colt from his shoulder holster and started with the first man to his left.

The dark eyes looking up at him radiated hatred. Even on his knees with his hands tied behind his back, the Vietnamese soldier projected unfiltered defiance.

The interrogator smirked. It was just what he was hoping for. Otherwise, he would've created it. This insolent soldier wasn't holding the big secrets—but the ones who did were watching.

The spook took his time. He trained at Langley to master precision theatrics, and this production was just getting started. He met the scowl looking up at him with an eerie, provocative smile and paused just long enough to evoke the response he was artfully co-constructing with his courageous victim.

In one fluid motion and surprising speed, he grabbed the prisoner by his dirty uniform collar and jerked him to his feet. He pressed the barrel of his pistol against the man's forehead. His incongruous smile hadn't shifted a millimeter.

The terrifying scene appeared utterly spontaneous, right down to his lack of surprise when the daring prisoner spat in his face. The sudden crack of his .45 startled everyone from both sides.

He lowered his smoking weapon and, with his other hand, calmly wiped the saliva from the bridge of his nose with a black bandana. He took a couple steps to his right and stood in front of the huddled figure next in line.

He trembled uncontrollably, grimacing hard to suppress his unruly nerves. He looked the spook in the eye, trying to ignore the pool of blood spreading towards his knees on the ground next to him. It took a moment, but he summoned the same scowl last worn by the now-lifeless pile beside him.

But this one found his voice. He started talking in Vietnamese, in hushed tones at first, but it rolled into an unconstrained tirade. One didn't need to understand the tonal language to know this wasn't the information they were after. His brazen protest was part of the show, so the interrogator allowed him to continue. The paymaster and highest-ranking officer were still two men down the line. They were so arranged for just this reason.

The spook shot a hard stare at the wide-eyed paymaster and slowed his movements for impact. His facial expression hardly shifted to signal what was coming. With an unsettling patience, he turned back towards the yammering man in front of him, inserted the barrel in his half-open mouth, and pulled the trigger. Somewhere in the middle of a sentence that didn't matter, the back of his head exploded.

It would have required nerves of steel not to talk after that. Nico recalled the rest of them spilled everything. The men on that intelligence gathering mission were decorated for the trove of information they captured that day.

Watching the macabre scene also required nerves of steel. By that time, Nico had long hardened up enough to feel victorious without getting caught in the morass that plagued less seasoned soldiers. The bush just didn't leave much room for morality. Not if you wanted to live.

Nico was focused on making it home. Being hard upped those odds, but he was also lucky; there had been many times he should have died for sure, and far too many others that his chances of survival stopped just short of none.

Nico recalled the very last mission those odds were pressed too far. Just two months into his second tour, he was on another LRRP mission walking point. He and his dog were moving fast. The enemy had picked up their trail and were in hard pursuit.

Known to the Vietnamese as the "men with green faces," the LRRPs were both hated and hunted. Because they were beating the guerrillas at their own game, they carried a bounty on their heads. They wore camouflage face paint to became one with the jungle and relied on stealth to prevent that blood money from being collected.

But this mission was different. Moving fast was anathema to LRRP tactics, but the priority was now evasion and exfiltration. In their hurry, one of the team lost their only compass. They used the sun and moon to navigate as best they could but their lack of precision and haste cost them. They were lost.

The team oscillated between navigation and evasion, struggling to stay ahead of their predators. The deadly chase went on for nearly two weeks. At headquarters, their trail went cold and the unit was officially designated as missing in action.

Back home, a sharply dressed officer reluctantly rang the doorbell of the family house. Nico's mother's heart skipped a beat when she opened the door to see him standing there in his pressed greens. She had tried to mentally brace herself for this moment when her son left for his first tour. However, she unraveled the moment she saw the solemn-faced Army officer. Her turmoil was too great to notice that he wasn't accompanied by a chaplain.

All Nico could think about was finding his way home. But he couldn't help but to curse himself for pressing his luck too far. During those agonizing days lost in the jungle, he made a promise to himself; if he got out of this one, he was done—he was going home.

The days melted into many. During one of them, Nico's dog alerted to something yet unseen in the jungle. He began barking. The LRRP team got low and froze. The nearby American infantry unit recognized the German Shepard's bark was far deeper than indigenous breeds. The dog located some friendlies. They had made it to safety.

Upon getting back to the fire support base, because of his MIA status, Nico's commanding officer granted him immediate leave and a ticket out. Nico was finally going home.

Every man in Vietnam dreamed of setting foot on the "freedom bird." But there was no immediate relief upon boarding the plane. There was only an unsteady silence driven by the pressure of being as "short" as one could get. And with that pressure came the fear—even then—of not making it out alive.

Men winced as the lumbering jet cleared the runway and began its slow climb. Only the drone of the engines filled the air as hundreds of survivors held their breath.

Upon clearing Vietnamese airspace, cheers broke out throughout the cabin. Unharnessed, ecstatic sounds of survival. They were going home.

⌒

Something was wrong. They had been circling over Guam too long and every veteran on the plane sensed the danger long before the staticky voice over the intercom announced it. Men cursed themselves for letting their guard down—they knew better.

The captain's announcement unleashed a torrent of pent-up frustration aimed at the faceless government who had risked their lives too many times. Lulling these men who sacrificed so much into celebration only to put death in front of them again was beyond cruel. Another static-riddled announcement crackled through the cabin.

Landing gear. The weapons of war failed to kill them: the bullets, the explosives, the booby traps, and the punji pits. They had also survived the land: the jungle, the leeches, the malaria, the snakes, the heat, and the endless rains of the monsoons. They survived it all. Damaged hydraulics were now trying to kill them.

In Vietnam, death often came quick. Many coped by surrendering to that destiny. The reasoning was simple; it was not worth worrying about because odds were that it would be over before they knew it. However, that fantasy crumbled against the gruesome reality. They knew there were endings far worse than sudden death. At 29,000 feet, they would have a veritable eternity to think about it.

The intercom was silent as the crew raced against the clock. The tension in the cabin ushered each man into the lonely corners of his mind. Some succumbed to fear. Others channeled it into the rage they had used to good effect in the field. The rest retreated into the familiar numbness of apathy. The plane continued to circle above the island airbase.

The men strained to decipher the rhythmic mechanical sounds now coming from beneath their feet. They felt their stomachs drop as the plane began a hurried descent. The entire cabin froze with another crackle of the intercom.

The landing gear was manually deployed and, judging from the tone the captain strained to keep steady, just in time. Rumors later circulated that they were coasting on the fumes of their reserve fuel tanks.

They were coming in fast. After urging his weary passengers to secure themselves for landing, the intercom abruptly cut out. That Nico cheated death once more was not the triumph it should have been. They landed just in time.

But fate wasn't done with him. On the next leg of his journey home, the plane's flaps weren't operating properly and once again, the captain came on to give the bad news.

Frayed men looked out the window at the western coastline of the mainland they never thought they would see again. Like prisoners peering through their cell windows, all they dreamed about sat tortuously beyond their reach.

Oakland's tower gave clearance for landing and dispatched emergency crews on standby to the runway. Whispered prayers wafted through the cabin....

...there are no atheists in foxholes....

Another treacherous landing was the final straw. Suppression collapsed into spasms of release. The clacking of seatbelts chattered throughout the cabin. Tearful men kissed the ground as the flood of raw emotion poured out onto their beloved American soil.

But they were coming home to a different America. The shaken returnees heard rumors of what was happening back home, but their naïveté landed in the epicenter of the spreading anti-war movement. Before their reluctant stateside handlers briefed them, the veterans could see it in their eyes. The news continued from bad to worse, cruelly yanking away the finish line of their war once more.

They could hardly believe their greeting. They were instructed to buy civilian clothes as soon as possible. Only days before their arrival at San Francisco International, a group of Hari Krishnas stabbed three returning soldiers bearing CIBs on their class A uniforms. This coveted badge signified that these men had been directly in the fight. Rather than being honored by their countrymen as they deserved, they were attacked.

Nico bought some civvies and got a bus ticket for the 2,000-mile trek home and tried to melt back into America. At the final bus terminal in St. Louis, he hailed a cab in the early morning light for the last leg of his journey to his family home—a place he had never thought he'd see again.

He requested a celebratory stop at White Castle where he bought breakfast for himself and his driver. The tiny burgers smothered in greasy onions never tasted so good. When the cabbie pulled up in front of the house, Nico froze.

He couldn't be sure how long he sat there; his eyes locked on his father's car in the driveway.

He reflected on the fifteen-year-old boy that walked out that kitchen door leading to the red-bricked carport when he left home for the last time. It seemed like a lifetime ago.

No—many lifetimes.

He felt the grief rising up from his core for that boy that was now gone forever. He caught the emotion in his throat and swallowed it down hard. The war finished the walls within him that his father started. Lost in this odyssey, he toggled back to the man he became since that day he walked out of his father's house.

The cabbie sat patiently looking at the weathered face with lost eyes in the rear-view mirror. It was the reflection of a man many times his age. A man who had seen too much. Done too much. Survived too much. The war eroded his features and chiseled away the boy who walked out of that door. A warrior was returning.

He didn't remember getting out of cab. Suddenly, Nico found himself at the threshold of the door in the carport. On the other side of it, he could hear muffled sounds of breakfast. His younger brother and sister would have left for school already. He paused as he placed his hand on the doorknob.

The weight of his olive drab duffle on his shoulder faded. The contact with the worn brass knob began a kaleidoscope of images and feelings as he fell backwards into his past again. He wasn't sure how long he stood there, but he returned just as he heard the cab slowly putter off behind him.

Nico took a deep breath, gently pushed the door open and was greeted by the smell of frying bacon before everything slowed.

From the doorway, his first image was the back of his mother as she stood over the stove. The pressed blue striped apron of his childhood sat in a perfect bow above her thin waist. He could tell from the length of the apron tie that she had lost too much weight since her son left for war.

As the door continued its slow, silent arc, his father's stern profile appeared. Quartering away from the door, he was seated at the table impatiently waiting for his breakfast. Though he could only see his one eye, it was enough. Nico had seen that penetrating look of disapproval a thousand times. He felt old anger stir his gut.

He took a step inside. The boy that left for war was gone. A man stepped over the door's threshold into the kitchen of his youth.

Nico didn't know about the recent house visit from the solemn-faced Army officer. He didn't know that the last his parents heard, he was classified missing in action and presumed dead. He didn't know that they believed they would never see Nico again. The Army had not bothered to let them know that he was alive. Or that their son was coming home.

And he didn't. Not the son that they remembered, anyway. That boy would forever remain lost in the jungles of Vietnam.

"I'm home!" Nico announced.

At the sound of his voice, his mother spun around with the skillet full of sizzling bacon in one hand and a spatula in the other. Her mouth froze open in silence. The skillet and spatula struck the hardwood floor with a metallic thud as her hands cupped her mouth to stifle her incredulous screams.

Before his startled father oriented to the unfolding scene behind him, his mother leapt at Nico. She embraced him with the full force of a desperate woman whose daily prayers were answered.

The tears of too many sleepless nights soaked into Nico's shirt. Her loud sobs filled his ears and for several moments, everything in the room was swallowed by the sheer power of a mother's love.

She wouldn't let go. And he didn't want her to.

Nico suddenly remembered that they were not alone. Between his mother's cries, his ears perked to something he had never heard before. He shifted to see past his mother's nestled head.

His father sat at the table, his head buried in those large hands, weeping.

17

Rolling Sanctuary

Driving a city bus was Ben's job, but it was much more than that.

To his regular passengers, he was the friendly and reassuringly familiar face they had known for decades. Some city residents literally grew up on his bus.

His forty-five years of service stood out as a durable constant in the uncertain urban landscape—places where it was hard to know who and what you could count on. Ben's route served some tough customers. His passengers watched him handle the regular disruptions that came from those trying to survive their urban jungle. In the city, violence and the streets wrapped around one another so tightly and so often, it hardly qualified as news anymore.

But they knew they could count on Ben: you could set your watch to his arrival. His sincere welcome greeted you at the opening door. Upon paying the fare, they sensed they were safe and protected in his mobile world—and they were. They noticed his watchful eyes toggle between the road and the rearward mirror reflecting their street-weathered faces. He *had* them ... and they knew it. However, the deeper truth was that the bus was also *his* sanctuary.

Ben had been brought up hard. A complicated family life left a broken home in its wake. At age three, he developed serious pneumonia and wasn't expected to live. His mother sent him to stay with his great grandmother in rural Arkansas. She took him in and raised him in a stark world where she taught the cardinal imperative—survival.

To him, his grandmother seemed just plain mean. As he grew older, he began to understand. She wasn't mean. She was just tough—and had to be—for them both. She knew all too well that growing up as a black man in America in the 1950s would require every stern lesson she could teach, and her version of love was delivered in just that way.

Ben took those lessons well. He had his first .22 rifle by the time he was six, and progressed to more powerful firearms as he grew older. He

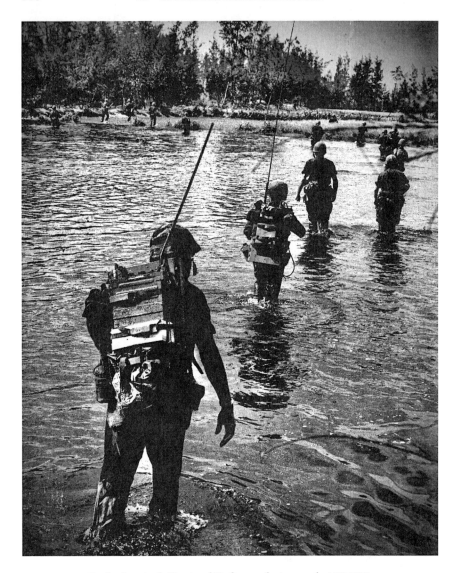

Soaked patrol. Dept. of Defense photograph A186108.

learned to shoot, hunt, and put food on the table. He learned the value of self-reliance and hard work. And he learned how to independently survive in a cold and inhospitable world that would not be offering him the benefit of the doubt. He would make his own way. And if there was a safe place out there for him, he would have to create it.

Ben came of age during the struggle for civil rights and the escalating war in Southeast Asia. The swift, chaotic current of both swept him up.

Like many poor young men of his generation, he found himself drafted into the Army destined for service in Vietnam.

And like the others, he didn't understand the war they made him fight in. They said he was going to save the world from the spread of communism. Ben was no stranger to being told by those in power how to see the world. Growing up in the South, his deference was expected and he was taught not to look them in the eye when they were saying it. The Army was no exception.

Being in the 4th Infantry in Vietnam was new and unforgiving, but because of his rugged upbringing, he was more prepared than most in boot camp. Ben knew how to go without, fend for himself, and survive when things got bad. He was also a natural rifleman. This quickly caught the attention of the Sergeant leading his squad. He needed replacements who knew how to shoot—it was their turn to go outside of the wire.

Ben's first patrol in the rice paddies was another typical day in Vietnam. That meant two things—it was hot and wet. The mission was simple—to look for VC and, if engaged, to kill them.

The primary problem with this imperative was that the enemy looked just like everyone else; the patrol was hunting for a needle in a muddy pile of needles. Unless one was caught red-handed wielding a weapon or carrying incriminating evidence, identifying the VC often relied on circumstantial information. To leadership, that was typically enough.

As the patrol made their way through the flooded rice fields, a Vietnamese youth spotted their approach and broke out into a run across the dry paddy dike.

Vietnam had seen war for a thousand years. One country after the next fought on their land, and the centuries built the survival of continuous warfare into the Vietnamese collective consciousness. To the peasant farmers, running from a group of armed men was instinctive. To an American soldier vigilant for an often unseen and un-uniformed enemy in this "free-fire zone," running suggested something else—guilt.

The Sergeant reflexively grabbed his best marksman.

"Shoot 'em!" he quickly commanded.

Ben never fired a weapon at another human being before. He anticipated that as an infantryman in war, the time would come when he would have to shoot at another man. But that decision was made already; he was bred to survive and if that's what it took to make it out of Vietnam, so be it.

In this guerrilla war, the enemy came in many forms. The Vietnamese were smaller framed, but he was not prepared to shoot at someone appearing so young. That wasn't supposed to matter to him—he was being given a direct order. But it did.

"Shoot! Now!!" the Sergeant urgently repeated.

Ben shouldered his rifle in mechanical compliance and easily found the small black-pajamaed blur through his aperture. The window of his moral impasse rapidly closed as the shrinking figure put distance between them. He instinctively tracked his target's movement through the sights like so many times before hunting rabbits back home. His awareness turned inward, his blinded muscle memory battling the eye of his conscious.

He vaguely heard the muffled yells of his squad leader, now outside of his cone of attention. It was only a matter of seconds but the mental duel was agonizing. Ben's finger tightened on the trigger.

The frames passed in slow motion by the time he made his decision. At the moment of truth, he steadily swung his rifle through the black blur and found the harmless outline of the paddy dike several feet in front of the fleeing youth. He squeezed off a single, well-aimed round.

The report of the rifle was overcome by a roaring concussion and fountain of erupting earth. The explosion swallowed the boy in a reddened cloud of laterite dust and smoke. The echo reverberated through the valley as the debris slowly rained down, splashing erratically in the surrounding paddy water.

Ben's muted haze suddenly broke to the loud cheers of his squad as the unexpected fireworks created a more dramatic moment of vengeance than anyone anticipated. Joy might have seemed oddly out of place ... unless one had lived in their boots.

Their jubilation was fueled by the pent-up frustrations of the many they lost to the trickery of the enemy's booby traps, and a local populace who never seemed to know who planted them in their fields. It was the cathartic release of men who, day after day, baked in sun looking for an elusive enemy, always themselves one step away from a similar fate.

"What goes around, comes around, Charlie! Xin Loi, motherfucker!"

What were the chances a single shot would find this buried enemy land mine? It happened so quickly, and the outcome so welcomed, the Sarge didn't seem to notice the intentionally pulled shot. He motioned to his RTO for the handset.

"We've got one enemy KIA, over," he proudly radioed back into base.

Ben stood frozen in disbelief. His brain numbly ran back the tape. He saw the boy running. He saw his sight picture. He saw the swing through his target, leading him by one meter. He saw the round strike precisely where he had intended. Then he saw the boy, in slow motion, disappear right before his eyes. The feelings began to breach his numbness.

Enemy? He was just a kid.

That day, Ben decided that he was never going to allow someone make him do the wrong thing again. Ever.

But the war was transforming them all. Once he would see for himself what all of the killing was about, he was no longer fighting to defeat communism. Ben resolved that no matter what the war sent his way, he would make his own choices. And he would fight to keep the two things he wasn't willing to lose—his life and his integrity.

However, Vietnam had a way of killing you even if you survived. Ben saw the randomness of cruelty meted out by both sides while in the field. He saw mortar rounds kill his friends only feet away from him while leaving him shaken, but unscathed. He saw plenty more bodies in civilian clothes who were assumed VC inflating the reports to a command hungry for body count.

The VC waged their own total war, terrorizing and killing a civilian population caught in the middle of their revolution. Each side claimed to be winning according to their own metrics. The planners believed they were right, so the slaughter continued. In Vietnam, no one was safe from anyone or anything for long.

And it wasn't only man-made death which was indiscriminate. When the VC weren't stalking you, the land did: the stifling heat, impenetrable jungles, swollen and swiftly moving streams, malaria-carrying mosquitoes, stinging ants, blood-sucking leaches, venomous snakes ... all knew you weren't of this place and hunted you because of it.

In Vietnam, even the heavens wanted you dead.

While on patrol during a torrential monsoon downpour, Ben's unit slowly moved through chest deep water of the rapidly filling rice paddies. The night sky was dramatically broken by crooked fingers of lightning streaking across the inky darkness. The saturated patrol held their rifles over their heads to escape the rising waters as they waded across, their weary bodies dragging their objective through the gauntlet of the night.

Suddenly, with a jolting crack, a glowing blue bolt searching for ground found the rifle barrel of the Sergeant leading the patrol. He limply sank into water as the jarring surge of energy dissipated through the column of stunned, water-logged men. The unforgettable smell of singed hair hung in the air.

Some men who arrived in Vietnam never left alive. Many who survived also never really left. To this day, Ben still felt the electric charge surge through his body whenever a midwestern thunderstorm rolled through, triggering the intruding film loop of the night a man was electrocuted only yards from him. That spark could then arc to any number of adjacent memories, waiting in his mind's que for something in his life close enough to rhyme with the war.

Or, it just might lie in wait, looking for an unoccupied mind at rest, its emptiness tempting the buried events that constant work and intense concentration helped keep in their shallow graves. Little did he know when he took the job that driving a bus would keep those memories buried, and become the refuge he was not yet aware he desperately needed.

Ben became a bus driver in the early 1970s and has been there ever since. It was his job, but it was much more than that. Though the bus belonged to the city, when he was behind the wheel, it was his—a rolling sanctuary for himself and his passengers. Though he didn't advertise his credentials, he lived the hard lessons about what was right and the integrity of protecting what was his in an unpredictable and predatory world.

Over the years, the city once touted as the gateway to the west descended into its own darkness of the soul, where one needn't do anything wrong to catch a bullet. Its decay commanded national attention as an epicenter of gang violence, record murder rates, racial tensions, and protests of abuses of power. In parts of the city, one was more likely to become a casualty than our troops stationed in overseas combat zones. And Ben's route ran right through the heart of it all.

Like the war in Vietnam, he couldn't control the city's boiling unrest surrounding his bus, but he had everything to do with what happened inside of it.

While behind the wheel, it was his realm to justly govern—his space to do what's right, and to help those in his community who relied on its shelter and secure passage. It was a place the weary could rest, get where they needed to go, and did so under a caring, watchful eye and steady hand. With many passengers whose safety depended upon his competence and sustained focus, his mind stayed securely tethered to the present.

And that was Ben's silent reward; there was no room for reflection. There was no room for the pain. At least not now.

There was only room to share the temporary refuge he created for them all to survive another day in the jungle, until the time came for them all to get off at their final stop.

18

Banana Cream Pie

He sat hunched over his desk staring at the dizzying spreadsheet of figures, the invisible grip of fear twisting through him.

For years after the war, Mac struggled to manage the anxiety that hijacked his body when he sensed peril. He learned to avoid the more obvious triggers, but it got tricky when the war showed up in the disguise of everyday life.

Though he owned his electrical contracting company for years, the recurrent terror of running out of what he needed to operate it would damn near paralyze him. As his business grew, so did the mounting stresses of making payroll and keeping the scales of money coming in and going out in balance. And his fear grew with it.

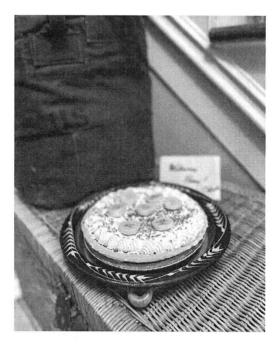

Mac had his own time-tested way of running his company, but his antiquated operations plan came with both a fiscal and emotional cost. That is why he finally hired a consulting firm, but their fees were much higher than anticipated. Now his balance sheet was in trouble. It was mistakes like this that he couldn't tolerate.

"It's all my fault," he

Author's photograph.

confessed in his psychotherapy session, cloaked in shame. It felt all too familiar and ran deep.

Way deeper than money.

What no one yet understood was how the fear of running out of necessities and of making critical mistakes activated his hidden war wounds. No one, including him.

Mac had suffered for years with severe headaches, anxiety, insomnia, and a recurrent nightmare of being overwhelmed by a mortal threat. Early in his therapy, we learned more about the terrifying dream.

"Doc, it's the same nightmare every time. I'm sitting on the porch of this rustic cabin looking out onto a wooded ridge in the mountains. All of a sudden, I see movement. Then I see the NVA come over the top of the ridge and begin pouring down the mountainside towards me. I don't have a weapon, any ammo, or what I need to defend myself." He would awake in a sweat, his head throbbing, with the terror of being overrun coursing through his veins.

In session, we connected the dots one by one.

The rustic porch in his dreamscape was his uncle's rural hunting cabin, a coveted refuge of his youth. However, this once-safe place was being invaded by the war.

My questions guided him through the murk of clues. The vista in the dream was familiar; he'd seen it twice before. The first time was from the porch of uncle's cabin which faced a ridgeline surrounded by the densely forested Ozark Mountains. Then it clicked for him; it was also the vantage of his entrenched position on Hill 881 where his Marine infantry unit was dug in during the siege of Khe Sanh in the winter of 1968.

From his position on that battle-scarred hilltop, he could see the mountains across the border into Laos. His combat unit lived and fought in those slit-trenched hills for months over some of the most viciously contested land in South Vietnam. Often, they did so without food, water, and running dangerously low on ammunition. The NVA wanted their high ground back and hurled all the men and ordnance they could muster to dislodge the embattled Marines.

Mac didn't think he would ever make it off that hill. In the face of the onslaught and the shortages, he confessed he used a fantasy to keep his will to survive intact.

"Doc, when things got the darkest for me on that hill, I would dream of making it home to eat my favorite dessert—my mom's banana cream pie. I would force myself to think about it and try to taste every bite. It gave me something to hold onto when it didn't look like I was going to make it."

If only he might live through another day to taste it once again. He sat entrenched in the sunbaked earth of his hell, imagining it's every scrumptious detail to drown out his grumbling stomach and parched throat. The fantasy didn't just distract his mind—it fed his soul as he wearily looked out upon those thickly forested mountains across the Laotian border.

As we sat in session that morning, we decoded the central, layered message of his dream: the war had taken the innocence and safety of his youth hostage, and didn't want to turn him loose. Because of this, he lived in fear of perpetual attack without the crucial supplies he needed to defend himself against what was coming.

We now understood how his well-founded fears of "running out" wired into his sense of impending annihilation. After these critical discoveries, something in him let go. The following session, he walked in the office, his face radiating glee.

"Doc, I can't believe it. I had the dream again. I'm on the porch like always, looking at that same ridge. But I feel differently. I feel calm, because when I see movement coming over the mountaintop this time, I don't see the enemy. It's deer that are running down it!"

He never had that nightmare again. The hunting cabin of his youth and sense of safety attached to that memory was finally restored.

Mac made other gains as his therapy progressed: he was feeling more peaceful, more self-assured, enjoying his marriage once again, and was methodically laying old issues and places he felt stuck to rest. The war's tight hold on him was loosening, and he was grateful. The following session, he came in beaming. "Doc, I've been searching my whole life to feel the way I do right now." His smile and testament were priceless.

The problem with trauma was, oftentimes it didn't stay that way. You are OK … until you aren't.

Just one month later, he felt the familiar grip of the past squeezing him—the fear of running out, of being in mortal danger because of it, and of making near-fatal mistakes. Those old convictions were reinserting themselves.

Big bills at work were coming due and he continued to tell himself how stupid he was to have hired the business consultants whose steep fees put him into what felt like a bottomless financial jam. By the time of his next session, the anxiety was smothering.

We started with his self-condemnation.

"Stupid mistakes you say … where had you felt that way before?" I inquired.

His fear of scarcity and annihilation was borne on Hill 881, but his self-flagellation for making mistakes was still buried. The calendar turned back rapidly as he started his search.

The first stop was childhood. Here he discovered the older messages he received from his father, a hardworking man who taught Mac many of the mechanical skills that would serve him so well later in his life. However, he was also liberal in his belittling comments. Eager to please his dad, Mac absorbed the criticism and simply tried harder. His work ethic benefited greatly. His self-esteem did not.

The years flipped forward to Vietnam. He related two memories not yet shared—experiences where mistakes were life or death.

"Yeah … it was a stupid mistake. By that time in my tour, I was a Corporal and a fireteam leader. We were going out on a 'killer team' patrol. These were four-man ambushes that would go out carrying only weapons and ammo—we travelled light. So instead of our packs and steel pots, we wore our soft covers. I wore this beanie I had bought from a villager for two packs of cigarettes. That Vietnamese hat barely fit my big head."

He brought me to the well-worn village footpath on which they set up their ambush that evening.

"It was dusk. We found a large granite boulder near a low stone wall that would offer good cover next to the trail leading to the village about 100 meters away. In front of us was a field and to our rear, a wood line. We were setting up. I was just putting in the blasting cap on the claymore mine when a burst of machine gun fire struck the ground only feet away. At first, I thought we were taking fire from a hooch in the village … but then I heard it."

Mac described looking up into the fading light and seeing the Huey helicopter circling around for another gun run. From cover, he started waving his arm to signal its crew to call off the attack. They were low enough that he could see the door gunner detect that movement and swing his M60 around to get back on target.

Mac's signaling was answered with a long burst of red tracers that began streaking from the descending bird right towards their position. Though the glowing line appeared like a near-continuous smear against the twilight, between every tracer round were four more rounds of 7.62mm ball ammo. Within seconds, the team's concealed ambush site was riddled with incoming rounds.

That they were all not killed was miraculous. Mac heard one of his men scream out as a bullet entered his calf. By the time he re-oriented toward the helicopter, his eyes widened further. A second helicopter had joined the hunt—a gunship. It was circling to bring its devastating armament of fixed machine guns and 2.75 inch high-explosive rocket pods to bear on their position.

"I then realized it was the beanie." Mac recounted. "I took it off and jumped out in front of the boulder waving my arms as the gunship lined up for a run on us. He must have finally realized we were Americans because they suddenly peeled off."

Mac's expression said it all as he closed the story. The wounded man lived, but the lesson was learned and the memory containing it seared into his mind.

"One little mistake nearly killed us all."

The puzzle of his current symptoms continued to fall into place.

A second event surfaced with the theme of mistakes and close calls. However, unlike many of his other days in Vietnam which were lost to the time-destroying grind of the war, he knew precisely when this next error happened. The reason he knew the exact day was because Mac was a base-ball fan.

His hometown Cardinals were playing the Detroit Tigers in the first game of the 1968 World Series. Bob Gibson had already struck out sixteen Detroit Tigers and was within one more of breaking Sandy Koufax's 1963 strikeout record.

No self-respecting Cardinals fan would dream of missing that game, even if you were at war halfway across the world. That Mac was on another nighttime killer team of four Marines lying in ambush somewhere in the jungle near Phú Bài was incidental; he would have been listening no matter where he was.

It was towards the end of his tour, so he was getting short. Because of that, he was willing to pull a double watch that night while the others slept. When a man was short and realized he might actually make it out alive, his nerves woke up after months of numbness that mercifully set in for a combat Marine ... if you lived long enough.

Because of that, the fear that greeted him when he first landed in Vietnam was now back. The closer he got to the end, the harder it was to sleep. Besides, he'd rather rely on his now–finely tuned battlefield senses than those of any other man—he was too close to returning home to leave anything to chance. By this point, he could almost taste it. He was going to have a slice of that pie again.

But the World Series beckoned another place and another time. The innocence of his childhood called to him. Mac melted into these two worlds as he stood watch over the darkened jungle trail, his earpiece plugged into his transistor radio. It was tuned into armed forces radio who was broadcasting the staticky daytime game live from the other side of the globe.

In one ear, he felt himself a boy again, back home brimming with excitement and anticipation as he listened to the crowd roar as the seven-teenth Detroit Tiger stepped up to the plate.

In his other ear were the now-fading sounds of creatures joining the jungle's nocturnal symphony. He felt the assuring weight of his M16 and the starlight scope in his lap which helped him sink further into the moment as the batter swung and missed the first two balls.

Mac's awareness of the trail dimmed, then vanished. He pictured himself in the speechless crowd back home as the pitcher wound up for his third pitch. An excruciating moment of silence broke to a deafening roar as jubilation filtered through the tiny earpiece. Gibson did it.

"YES!!" Mac heard himself yell out reflexively, the sound crashing into the stillness of the jungle night.

His attention snapped back as he froze. Holding his breath, he strained in the darkness to figure out if he had actually made that noise or if he simply imagined he had.

His uncertainty was broken by the faint sound of rustling leaves. He zeroed in on the disturbance in the darkness. The movement was directly in front of his position.

His pulse quickened as he placed his hand on his weapon while silently raising the starlight scope. It turned the dark jungle into hues of illuminated yellows and greens. As he peered into the scope, the hair on the back of his neck stood up as his primordial instincts reacted.

Two green eyes were staring directly at him.

Time melted away as each creature sat motionless, sizing up the other.

The eyes slowly shifted position and revealed a partial outline. The movements were feral and fluid—this was no man. A moment later, its silhouette emerged into the starlight scope's field of view.

Mac gripped his M16 a little tighter before the large black panther that was stalking him sensed the lost element of surprise and silently vanished into the thick underbrush. All that was left to testify to the near-death encounter was a single swaying palm frond.

Mac let out a labored exhale in session, echoing this close call in the jungle five decades earlier. Their small team's camouflaged position in enemy territory was their primary defense. As a seasoned team leader, he was well aware of the potentially fatal mistake of giving away that position. No one was hurt, but the error now forever encoded.

And that was precisely the problem. His mind and body wouldn't let him forget the lesson. In Vietnam, a mistake—any mistake, could be your last. He couldn't afford to make a fatal misstep or imagine where the cost could be anything less.

Because to him, it was *all* life or death. Or at least it felt that way. It was no longer a decision, but instinctual. The body had kept score.

In session that day, he uncovered this old lesson. He now understood how his fear of making a mistake reached so deeply. He recognized that his business was not life or death, even though it felt as though it were. But rather than heralding his physical death, finding those buried fears started the process of releasing him....

...releasing himself from the past. Welcoming him to the present as a man capable of error without anyone dying. One who could afford the grace of imperfection without berating himself. One who could enjoy the freedom of being human without the lurking fear of annihilation.

And it affirmed the man he is....

...a man who had worked so hard to feel good about who he was, mistakes and all. It was the reward he had been living for all this time and didn't even know it.

⁓

With his dress greens on and his sea bag slung over his shoulder, Mac made a call halfway across the world, and listened with anticipation to the staticky ringtones. He had not heard her voice for thirteen months. His war was over. He was calling to tell his mother that he was coming home.

It was waiting for him when he walked through the door of the childhood home that he thought he would never set foot in again. Her banana cream pie had never tasted so good.

19

Champ

He's always been a champion. Though he earned that title in the boxing ring, the nickname bestowed to him by fellow black Marines was shortened to "Champ." And due to a racist in his combat outfit, it settled on "Chimp." Nicknames in Vietnam weren't always flattering or fair, but when they stuck, they stuck.

Not that Ramey was any stranger to racial hatred. Growing up in St.

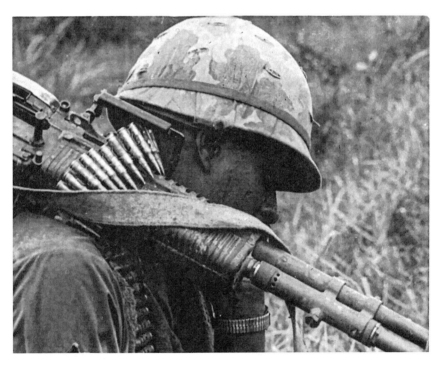

M60 gunner. National Archives, photograph 111-CCV-591-SC662111 by Sp4 Christopher Brow.

Louis in the 1950s landed him squarely in the middle of a deeply divided country. Ramey absorbed the bitter lessons that black parents taught their children in order to navigate a culture that still denied them the freedom bestowed upon them almost 100 years earlier. But with the new decade came fresh hope.

So many worked for this hard-fought run at equality, and finally, it arrived. Ramey recalled when the Civil Rights Act of 1964 became law. He and his girlfriend celebrated the landmark legislation by going to a restaurant downtown that only a day before was off limits to black patrons.

Ramey scanned the dining room. Disapproving white expressions said what the silence wouldn't, and returned to their meals. An elderly black couple seated by the window greeted their uncomfortable entry with a quiet, pained embrace. Ramey waited for several unanswered minutes before they seated themselves at a lonely two-top in the corner.

The world in that room made them as invisible as they felt. They watched as the staff and other diners did their best to go about their lives in denial of the freshly inked law of the land. With a hurried stride, the waitress walked back and forth by their table. Her resentment chiseled the muscles of her face and kept her eyes locked straight ahead as she made yet another pass.

"Excuse me. May we have some menus?" Ramey steadily asked.

She stopped dead in her tracks with the unapologetic nerve not to even pretend to be surprised by her neglect. She placed a self-righteous hand on her hip, and shot him a penetrating stare to punish him for halting her charade. Ramey didn't back down. He was never one to walk away from a necessary fight.

The waitress made no effort to hide her contempt. She retrieved two menus from the caddy at the hostess stand by the door and stormed over to throw them down on the table before spinning away without a word. She had barely completed her hasty pivot when Ramey spoke up again.

"And we would like some water, please."

Ramey watched her every movement hemorrhage just a little of a lifetime of hatred. When she returned carrying two partially filled water glasses, he instinctively leaned into the wall behind him. Taking his cue, his girlfriend winced to brace herself.

The sound of the glasses slamming into the wooden tabletop startled nearly everyone in the room. All looked shocked by the disturbance. Everyone but the elderly black couple, their faces etched with a pain that only they could know. The impact sent water all over the paper menus and the seated couples' sleeves. Satisfied she finally made her point, the waitress slowly walked off with a smirk, taking a casual lap through the dining room as if to bask in the collective silent appreciation of her patronage.

Ramey got the message: you could legislate the rules, but not the heart. While it was their right to eat there, he had too much self-respect to subject them both to scorn just because some politicians now said they could eat anywhere they wished.

While Ramey wasn't welcome to have lunch with white folks, they didn't seem to mind if he served in their military or fought in their country's wars. At least on paper.

Less than two years later, Ramey joined the United States Marine Corps. He graduated from high school on a hot midwestern Friday in June and left for boot camp that following Monday. Ramey wanted to box for the Corps. Vietnam derailed that dream. They needed him elsewhere.

After eight weeks, he became a Marine with an MOS of 0331; though Ramey had always been a fighter, he was now a M60 machine gunner. By November of 1966, Ramey set foot in Vietnam with 2/9th of the 3rd Marine Division, whose moniker "Hell in a Helmet" foreshadowed what was coming.

True to their motto, they were the first to fight and did so in the most viciously contested property that separated this partitioned war-torn country. Ramey was sent to the same place as the rest of the Marines in Vietnam—I Corps.

This "demilitarized zone," or DMZ, was shameless in its lie; it became the epicenter of the war. Golf Company was one of many Marine combat units spread across the DMZ separated by the Bến Hải River as the first line of defense against communist aggression against South Vietnam. Even now, Ramey can still hear the recurring urgent call that he was needed in the fight.

"Guns up!!"

And Ramey was in the fight a lot. The 2nd Battalion of the 9th Marine regiment saw sustained combat throughout late 1966 and 1967. One day in July, his Commanding Officer summoned him to report to his command post. This couldn't be good.

As he hustled the CP, his mind swam with a hundred imagined infractions, none of which he could remember violating. He regretted that he was right—he wasn't in trouble. A Red Cross notice was waiting.

While Ramey was trying to survive combat in southeast Asia, his brother fell prey to the war back home on the tough urban streets of St. Louis. He was granted emergency leave to return stateside for the funeral. With his orders in hand, he reported to Đà Nẵng airfield.

The loadmaster of the Military Airlift Command confirmed Ramey's name on the flight manifest, and waved him aboard. As the rear gate of the cavernous C130E transport plane yawned open, he started up the ramp before freezing in his tracks. He stood silently for a moment to make sure what he was seeing was real. In the cargo bay of the plane lay twenty-two symmetrically arranged rectangular aluminum boxes.

With nine months of intense guerrilla warfare, Ramey saw plenty of dead bodies. Too many. But this was different. They were his only company for the excruciating twenty-two-hour flight to Travis Air Force base in California. He was going home to pay respects to his dead brother with the remains of his fellow fallen brothers in arms on their final trip out of the bush. Without any distractions, he couldn't help but to stare at those silver boxes in a ceaseless present. He would forever cringe at the number twenty-two.

It was July 29, 1967. While Ramey was confined in his own hell, the 2/9th would soon find theirs again. The 3rd Marines was launching Operation Kingfisher. Ramey's unit was part of this larger effort to block the NVA from infiltrating into eastern Quảng Tri province. The Marines came loaded for a big fight and planned on hitting Charlie hard. Accompanied by M48 tanks and other armor, they pushed north along Route 606 to intercept the enemy.

The NVA didn't give the Marines the fight they wanted. After making no contact that night, at sunrise, the empty-handed Marines started back to their lines. But their ponderous show of offensive strength became their weakness.

The tanks were too big and too heavy to take an alternate route back; the adjacent roads and bridges wouldn't support them. Because of this, the Marines were forced to violate what everyone who preceded them in this guerrilla war learned the hard way—never use the same trail twice.

The command-detonated mine opened the attack, the explosion instantly wounding five Marines. Another mine struck the rear of the column followed by smothering automatic and mortar fire on those trapped in the kill zone. Rocket propelled grenades struck the armored vehicles, their shaped charges penetrating the armor plating and showering the encased marines with molten shrapnel. The combined-arms ambush used every principle of fighting the communists similarly learned the hard way.

The Vietnamese learned to grab their enemy "by the belt"; it was their tactic for getting in close to their targets to negate American air and artillery superiority. The Marines were under withering small arms fire. A risky but devastating danger-close napalm attack eventually broke the enemy's grip on the embattled Marine positions. The day's heavy fighting resulted in twenty-three Marines killed and 253 wounded.

Ramey did not know that fate had saved him from being one of those twenty-three killed. After the funeral, upon returning to his unit and learning what happened, he couldn't be grateful that he was spared. The guilt wouldn't let him.

Like Ramey, Lance Corporal Larry Kinard was a machine gunner. Like Ramey, Larry was a boxer. He was also Ramey's friend. That fateful day, he was Ramey's replacement on this mission as a rear-guard gunner. On Operation Kingfisher, Larry was shot six times and was one of the twenty-three Marines slain that day. Larry hailed from Philadelphia, the city of brotherly love. On July 29, 1967, Ramey lost two brothers.

For years, Ramey suffered from relentless nightmares depicting his impossible dilemma, the powerlessness, and the immense loss of that day. In the dream, he sees himself being sent down to the river on a water run from his company's elevated, dug-in positions. When he returns with the filled water bladders and canteens, there is an eerie silence on the hill. He sees no one and enters their unmanned perimeter without the challenge of those who should have been on watch. He calls out to his fellow Marines but there is no reply. He searches until he sees a large bomb crater up ahead. He cautiously approaches the crater and peers over the edge. In the hole are the dead bodies of all of his comrades in arms. He would wake up with a start, the sweat soaking the pillow beneath him.

The next time Ramey set foot on American soil, he had endured thirteen months of intense combat. Fresh from the war, the righteous fight and being of service to others was in Ramey's blood. He came home forever changed but necessity required that he move on. He needed a job and wanted to continue in service. But he also wanted to box.

Later in his life, he transitioned from professional boxer to head coach, and invested his heart, wisdom, and talent into the struggling young men and boys in his community. Though he had not yet connected the dots, Ramey was trying to save these youth from the carnivorous streets that had taken his brother from him. He would give them a refuge, teach them how to fight for the right reasons, and how to defend themselves from the indifference of a world that would not be looking out for them. But after his discharge from the Marine Corps, he would first have to look out for himself.

The ailing American economy didn't leave many options for returning veterans, but law enforcement offered a natural transition. He didn't expect the city changed its deep racial animus while he was overseas and wasn't surprised when he found the same obstacles upon his return. Then again, to the public, serving your country in Vietnam with honor and distinction didn't count for much no matter your skin color.

Because of these walls, Ramey only tried harder. He wanted to become a cop and fought for the right to be one no matter what America thought of him. At least that was the way he looked at it. Ramey graduated the training academy and joined the Metropolitan Police Department.

He felt right being in unform again, but Vietnam tore away any illusions about the way things worked in the world.

On one of his first domestic calls, he and his partner confirmed the address before ringing the doorbell. A short, frail elderly woman answered the door. She pushed her horn-rimmed glasses up her nose before squinting to make eye contact. Ramey smiled at the endearing image of the delicate matriarch.

"Good afternoon, Ma'am. Did you call for the police?"

"Yes … but I didn't call for two niggers."

That delicate face soured as she stepped back and slowly closed the door before the sound of the deadbolt clicked firmly into place.

It didn't go any better with some of his fellow officers and leadership. His Sergeant was watching his every move. While on street duty, Ramey observed a cute blond in a convertible commit a minor traffic violation. He didn't stop her, but within fifteen seconds, his supervisor pulled up behind him and instructed the rookie to join him in his cruiser. He confronted him for harassing the white woman and when Ramey told him the truth, the Sergeant accused him of lying.

"Sarge, you're not important enough for me to lie to." Ramey looked him right in the eye and got out of the car. After that, it was on.

And it wasn't just the racism. The city PD was infested with moral rot. Ramey struggled with the abuse of power and misdeeds of both white and black colleagues. The final straw was the unethical actions of a fellow black officer. After that, he began hunting for a transfer. When it came to what was right, Ramey didn't give a damn what color you were.

He considered himself lucky to land a trooper position with the State Highway Patrol, only to find human darkness continued to follow him. His first meeting in the capital city with his new supervisory Sergeant immediately cast a shadow on the future Ramey hoped would be better.

They stood staring at one another for several moments without a word passing between them. Without interrupting his intense gaze, his supervisor cocked his head and was the first to break the strained silence.

"Ya know…."

Ramey waited for him to complete his statement after another pause which lasted almost as long as his glare.

"…there's a whole bunch of rednecks in Jefferson City…."

"…and I'm one ova 'em."

Ramey didn't give the Sergeant an inch of the response he was looking for. He also wasn't surprised when the rumors filtered down; that Sergeant was an unapologetic member of the local chapter of the Ku Klux Klan. Ramey endured one indignity after the next under the thumb of his supervisor. Like all of the insults that came before, Ramey channeled the vitriol into his drive to do better and be better.

In spite of that, he liked being a trooper. But it kept getting harder. It wasn't just the hate; the war started revisiting him more often and the pressure kept rising. The nightmares and sleepless nights squeezed from one side; the intensity of his job pushed on the other. The violence, the car wrecks, the suicides, the mangled bodies. It just didn't stop. The end of his law enforcement career couldn't come soon enough. Just three days before his retirement date, his hateful supervisor died, and with that announcement, a grant of seventy-two hours of peace.

After he retired, Ramey didn't waste another minute with those looking to tear others down. His passion was building others up. He had spent so much of his life fighting: in the ring, in the jungle, and on the streets and highways.

He invested much of his newfound time and energy into his role as a boxing coach working with urban youth—showing them there was another way out: a way out of poverty. A way out of the dead-end streets. A way out of the gangs. A way out of being treated as less-than. And a way into fighting for something worth believing in—themselves. Ramey was finally back in the ring where he belonged, where he reclaimed his title.

Showing them how to be a champ.

Epilogue: Like many returning war veterans, Ramey faced many challenges reintegrating back into society, and did so facing prejudices of many types. Ramey's dream was to box for the Marine Corps and beyond. The war interrupted that ambition, but in spite of the obstacles he faced carrying his war trauma, fighting racial prejudice and ostracism as a returning Vietnam veteran, he regained his title of "champ." He eventually became a head coach and trainer for urban youth and helped hundreds of kids compete in national boxing leagues. Sadly, he lost some of his fighters to the violent streets from which he was attempting to protect them. Like many veterans, his dedication to mentoring and helping others became an integral part of his search for resolution, peace, and trauma recovery.

20

The Grenade

Marvin had been back from his healing and reconciliation trip to Vietnam sponsored by the Soldier's Heart organization for a couple of months now.

He continued to marvel as to how his journey unfolded—the utter serendipity of the many connections he made with others and with his past.

"My head is just swirling still," he said. "If you would have asked me before I left to write down the list of wishes for all that I got out going back to Vietnam, I could have never done it."

During the war, Marvin was an infantry squad leader with the 5/60th,

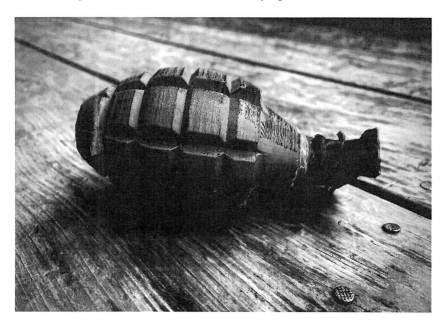

Author's photograph.

9th Infantry Division. His tour ended when his point man's boot pressed into the nearly invisible wire stretched across the jungle trail. Had Marvin not looked down at that precise moment, he would not have survived to make that trip back to Vietnam in 2017—he would have never left the country alive the first time.

The trip wire triggered a booby-trapped grenade which riddled his right arm, hip, and pelvis with shrapnel, and took one of his fingers.

As bad as it was, it could have been worse. The grenade blast also peppered his helmet with fragments—fragments that would have hit his face had he not been looking down as he tried to free his boots from the tangle of jungle vines. While the medic treated his injuries, his squad mate showed him the tattered helmet that spared his life and started his long journey of recovery from his physical and emotional scars.

This traumatic event was the impetus for a spider web of interlocking events and emotional pitfalls that persistently revisited him later in life. Our therapy sessions peeled back the layers of those wounds.

"I had this crazy combat dream last night," he said.

"Crazy how?" I ask.

Marvin narrated his repetitive nightmare—the incubus that first visited him on December 26, 1968, while on convalescent leave at Fitzsimmons Army Hospital.

"I'm always in a hooch. A grenade rolls in. I look for an egress—an opportunity to get rid of it, but every time I turn towards a window or door to throw it out, it closes or disappears. I can't get away from it. I try to take cover in the corner but the floor tilts and rolls it towards me, first along the mud floor, but then the floor changes to wood and I can hear the distinctive sound it makes as the grenade slowly rolls towards me along the floor. Clunk.... Clunk.... Clunk.... I then wake up screaming."

This recurrent nightmare, he relates, was typically in color and always the same, but last night's dream was very different:

"Everything is in black and white. We are on a military bus. I'm with others I know, but I don't know exactly who, and I am my current age. A grenade comes in through the window. My head says to stay in cover, behind the seat with its protective metal back and pad. It doesn't explode and I know it's a delayed fuse, but I don't know how long the delay is. My heart tells me to move towards it and before my head tells me not to, I pick it up and then throw it out the window. This time, the window doesn't close or disappear and we are OK—we are finally safe."

Marvin sits looking baffled, but curious by what he just shared.

We start exploring the different details of the dream. It unraveled in layers of meaning. We filled in the external pieces of the details like the edges of a jigsaw puzzle—who the people were, what he saw, thought, and felt. As he projected himself into the nightmare and began to narrate, a portrait of the dream became a living three-dimensional presence in the room.

"I somehow know them—the others in the dream, yet I don't know who all of them are. I should be staying in cover but I don't ... against my better judgment, I move towards the grenade."

"And what type of man does that ... leaves the safety of cover to retrieve a live grenade to protect himself and others?"

His eyes closed as he searched for answers—and they kept coming.

"Hmmm ... a selfless man ... a ... well ... it doesn't fit me, but ... a heroic man...."

"Heroic?"

"Well, I'm not that—I don't like that term, but yeah...."

"You judge that you are not heroic ... perhaps ... perhaps a courageous man?"

"Yeah ... that fits better than heroic."

"I'd like you to focus on the grenade. Tell me about it."

"It's an old WWII pineapple style grenade, not the kind we had in 'Nam. In the dream, it is the color of a dark metallic object like you would see in an old black and white movie...."

I track, reflect, and interpret as we moved through the narrative.

"So somewhat out of place in the present. Not the type you actually used in the war. So, it's old...."

"Yeah, old. I can see the hole through the top where the pin used to be."

"I'd like you to take notice of that grenade and I want you not to think about it, but to drop down into your heart and just notice what that grenade means. What is it saying to you?"

He responds easily and simply, "Fear—it is something to be feared."

"Yes ... an old fear," I remark as I knit the two interlocking pieces together for him.

Silence....

"I'd like you to try something. I'd like you to try to become one with the grenade. Go inside of it. What do you notice? Be open to what it may have to tell you."

His eyes are closed, but within a few moments of quiet reflection, a wry smile of recognition slowly spreads across his face.

"It's weird. When I go inside of it, I feel calm ... peace." He pauses again and the smile melts away.

"Now it's trying to resist me going inside of it. It keeps wanting to come into me versus me going into it. There is still something in my guts ... it's churning ... something still there."

"So when you face it—go inside of it, you find calm and peace. But when it goes inside of you, you feel something churning in you, maybe that fear you mentioned...."

I studied Marvin's silent facial reactions to the interpretation carefully, wondering if it landed.

He paused and then a physical shudder went through his body like an electrical current searching for ground. In the next moment, the smile partially reappeared.

"Feels like something—I'm not sure what—but something just left. A burden maybe."

He sat quietly as the puzzle pieces continued to rotate in his mind until they found their partnering edge, and then joined. He opened his eyes signaling both a shift and the completion of his journey inward. There was a noticeable, but indescribable difference in the light shining through his eyes.

We processed what he just experienced. With guided questioning, he created a narration of where and what he just visited and the wisdom he retrieved from the depths of his wounds. Together, we constructed the log of his journey.

We started at the trailhead of the notable physical shift and descended into his past. He arrived back at the shudder. It was unmistakable; something painful, a burden he carried for most of his life, left his soul.

The dream was just the first waypoint. The stubbornly entrenched nightmare held his inescapable terror of the chi-com grenade that changed his body and life forever. But the trail continued far beyond the dream.

The tapestry of Marvin's life and the insights he retrieved knitted themselves together by unseen hands. He dug deeper and revealed rich layers of meaning, which simultaneously told the story his wounded warrior and his current adult self striving to recover from his war trauma. He finally acknowledged his courage during the war, and the courage he reclaimed when he went back to Vietnam exactly fifty years later to face his old fears, to look his former enemy in the eye, and to heal.

This is what the bus full of people in his dream represented; it was the vehicle he and fellow travelers with Soldier's Heart used during his pilgrimage back to Vietnam. That bus drove him to the South Vietnamese Delta, the very earth on which he was forever changed. He searched for several sacred places he needed to revisit and, against the odds, found them; none of the sites were marked as the Vietnamese spared no effort wiping the remnants of the American War from the landscape.

Marvin discovered them by trusting his gut to find his way, just as the young squad leader had so many years earlier. Instinct and synchronicity merged, not once, but several times.

With the help of a local farmer, Marvin found Firebase Moore where his high school classmate and best friend in Vietnam, Ronnie Powers, was killed by a short mortar round less than one month into his tour. Once he knew he was in the right place, Marvin reached into his pocket. He pulled out his harmonica which traveled 8,000 miles for that very moment, and on that hallowed ground, played "Taps" for Ronnie.

Marvin then traveled to Rạch Kiến and found the century-old French farmhouse where his point man tripped the booby-trapped grenade. Finally, and almost unbelievably, he met and befriended a former VC soldier, Tầm Tiền, whom he fought on the very same battlefield on September 26–27, 1968, in the Plain of Reeds. The old battle-scarred foes smiled and marveled at their reunion, this time in peace. Marvin traveled back to Vietnam with trepidation to face his trauma, and brought back healing he couldn't have imagined.

And last night, in a terrifying nightmare, Marvin trusted his heart, mastered his fear, and threw it all out of a window which, this time ... finally ... didn't disappear.

~

Epilogue: Marvin first experienced the "grenade" nightmare on December 26, 1968, and it plagued him for decades. He had the variant of this terrifying dream about fifty years later just before his session work described in the above story. After this transformative experience, he purchased a ceramic "grenade" mug, closely resembling the grenade that wounded him, from a local veteran-owned coffee company. Now he starts each day with a cup of coffee from this mug. In his words, "I now feel like I own the grenade rather than the grenade owning me." He never had the nightmare again.

21

Father's Map

This wasn't Don's first existential threat. Ever since the war, he's been waiting for the other shoe to drop. When it did, it fell on the entire planet.

The governor's shelter-in-place orders during the Coronavirus Pandemic of 2020 provided the perfect opportunity to tackle long-overdue projects around the house. Cleaning out his over-stuffed garage was next. But his stamina wasn't what it used to be. Don figured he'd start this daunting job with the most densely packed corner while he was still fresh.

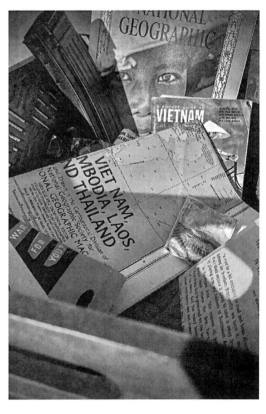

Don was no newcomer to cleaning out a garage bulging with the accumulated wares of a man's life. In his family lineage, that job always fell to the oldest surviving son. Boxes were stacked from floor to ceiling. He had planned for the next crisis for so long, he forgot what was there. He also didn't anticipate the journey into his past laying before him.

As he disassembled the precarious mountain, he caught a glimpse of the

Author's photograph.

nostalgic faded blue and red logo. Buried for years, he smiled with its fresh discovery. He recognized the old wooden beer crate immediately.

The Point Beer Brewery hailed from Stevens Point, Wisconsin. It was founded just a couple of years before the outbreak of the Civil War and supplied beer to the war weary union troops. It was also Don's father's favorite brand.

Beer was a big deal in many ethnic enclaves of St. Louis, but none more than the German community. Don's family lived in the heart of it and had a proud tradition of hard work, technical skills, and service. They also played hard and after their long workdays, enjoyed many cold steins at the local tavern.

As war clouds gathered on the twentieth-century European horizon for the second time, FBI agents started showing up at the corner bar. Their watchful eyes, government suits, and feeble efforts to blend into the tight knit community made them all the more conspicuous.

It was obvious to all—they were monitoring German patrons for signs of subversive activity. When war broke out in 1941 with Japan and then Germany, Don's uncles and most other neighborhood men immediately joined the service. The feds' visits to their bar became fewer and further between.

In the wake of Roosevelt's famous declaration of war speech, Americans from all over the nation reported in droves to induction centers. Some years earlier, Don's father lost a couple of fingers and severely damaged his hand while operating a punch press. His father continued the war effort as a stateside machinist but was classified "4F" and deemed ineligible for service due to those injuries. While he would never have to go to war, his son was not so lucky.

Like many young men of his generation, Don was drafted into service to fight in Vietnam. And like many who fought and died there, he couldn't find Vietnam on a map before his deployment. He only knew that his country had called, and he was going to answer no matter where it took him.

When he arrived in Vietnam, Don quickly figured out that knowing where one was being sent was important.

Life and death important.

On his first trip to the bush, he learned that locations carried crucial information about the fate of those sent there. He noticed the expressions of those who processed his orders.

These were men who knew what the names of those destinations on the map of southern Vietnam meant. Their faces told the silent story of places many young Americans were sent and never returned from.

As the helicopter leapfrogged from one outpost to the next, Don quickly gathered whatever information he could from the base's garrison.

The closer he came to his assigned company area, the more ominous the facial reactions became. Their eyes said what their mouths wouldn't. Don mentally plotted his path into the gorge of the war's uncertainty.

Don filed the names of these places away. The survival value they provided was critical—enough to remember the indecipherable names in the tonal language that didn't come easy to American ears. He would jot them into his letter writing materials when the time presented itself to keep those at home appraised of his movements. Better to know what's coming than not. Oddly, he found bad news was better than the darkness of his fearful imagination.

In war, enlisted men lived in this uncertainty until someone with more power decided they needed to know something. As the information trickled down the ranks, it was cloaked in sterile operational terms—words that conveyed only a limited peek into their future.

It was the only glimpse Don was supposed to have. Like the C-rations that were just enough to keep a weary fighting man combat-ready, it was never enough to satisfy their hunger—painful pangs for the truth that no one seemed to want to acknowledge or deliver. In a war beset by lies, a man needed to know—know a truth he could count on.

But the truth was everywhere. Don just needed to learn where to find it.

It was there in the dull sounds of war in the distance, the stench of decay in the air, and the black body bags laying off to the side of the helipad waiting for their final ride out of the bush.

Men lie. His eyes couldn't.

A soldier had to develop a chest of tools to cope with the immense strain of war's violence. To stave off the suffocating despair, Don dreamed of seeing home again. But when he finally returned in October of 1969, all he found was the house he grew up in. And when he got there, nothing was the same.

The horror of what Don experienced as an infantryman operating in the Central Highlands was unforgettable. But it wasn't for lack of trying. Indeed, that was the problem. He did everything he could to put the war behind him. But the unforgettable wouldn't stay in the past. His father could see the truth in his eyes—this was not the same young man he reluctantly watched go off to war.

And it was no secret that Don and his father struggled in their relationship ever since his return. His father tried to talk to his son many times about the war, but Don just couldn't go there—the wound was too deep and too fresh.

Don couldn't address the war because he didn't know how. It was easier to see fault within his father, so he told himself that no one cared.

Though his father was an old staunch German who hadn't seen war and wouldn't understand, it wasn't that he didn't care. Quite the opposite. Maybe he cared too much. And that further drove the wedge between them.

Don kept his inquisitive father at bay with irritable posturing. Like a territorial dog, he would snap at his father's overtures when they got too close. When those warnings stopped working, Don packed up and left his father's home for the final time.

Striking out on his own took him down some hard roads, but they all paled in comparison to the one he was avoiding. He didn't realize the war's shadow he was trying to evade would follow him no matter how far he was from home.

For years, their relationship followed the angular contours of their physical separation. Don and his father occasionally tried to talk but each effort was doomed before it started. There was too much that they couldn't talk about that got in the way of what little they could.

The day President Nixon resigned from office, Don picked up the phone. He knew his father's politics and that the news would come as a blow to his conservative leanings. He barely completed his sentence when he heard his father hang up on him.

"It's your son. I told you the guy was a crook...."

They careened apart and never recovered. Then, they ran out of time.

As the eldest son, in the wake of his father's death, it was his job to empty the family house. Because of their schism, Don went about this disposal task without the headwind of sentimentality.

As a survivor of the Great Depression, his father rarely threw anything away. They at least had that in common. A week after the funeral, Don stood staring at the tightly packed garage not knowing where to begin.

Stoic piles eventually formed on the concrete floor. Some could be sold, but the largest mounds were destined for donations or the land fill. There were but a few things Don wanted for himself.

One was the dusty Point Beer crate he found tucked in the back of the wall of storage shelves holding his father's vast collection of tools.

In that crate, Don came across patinaed keepsakes such as antique skeleton key locks and other collectibles signaling a man fascinated with a well-machined piece of steel. However, it was the misplaced large manila envelope that caught his attention.

He carefully turned it over and recognized his father's steeply sloped penmanship. His heart sank before his mind finished reading the word.

It simply read "Vietnam."

At the time, Don couldn't bring himself to open it. Even the word sent a paralyzing shockwave through him. The anxiety doused any spark of curiosity—he didn't want to go there. He quickly looked away to anchor his thoughts in the presence of the dimly lit garage.

He took a deep breath and felt its emotional grip loosen. He solemnly tucked the sealed envelope back into the Point Beer crate that was going home with him.

Another time, he told himself. There was just too much left to do.

But he knew that was a lie. The truth was that there was never a good time to think about Vietnam, much less talk about it. For decades, he worked hard to master sidestepping the war.

Over time, these efforts bore diminishing returns. He took a job and settled in Chicago to put distance between him and his family. Then the distraction of his job stopped working. Alcohol worked for a while, but the war patiently waited for him on the other side of its numb respite.

Eventually, nothing hid the truth he was being pushed towards. The nightmares were getting worse, and that required more alcohol to quell them. Out of options, he finally surrendered and went to get help.

Maybe that was why he found that old beer crate twenty-five years after his father's death while cleaning out his own garage. He was in a different place now. Maybe he was ready to find it.

Don spent the intervening years working hard on the many war scars within him. He developed some compassion for himself and, in so doing, began to reconstruct his jagged narrative of the war. He struggled to put together the shards of memories into a coherent story. He cried and grieved. He communalized secrets, the horror and the trap of impossible life and death choices with no good outcomes. He honored the pain and its reasons for being there.

Finally, Don began to heal.

So, when he found the manila envelope during the pandemic of 2020, he only paused … before he carefully opened the deteriorated glue seal. The mystery of its contents brought a flurry of feelings out of the depths of his gut….

…but this time, he kept going. He was done running.

Don carefully reached inside and felt the stiff paper stock. By touch, it wasn't what he expected, and his curiosity urged him to pull the first glimpse far enough out of the envelope for a hint.

Below the pale border, he saw topographical shades of sage green and hued elevations cordoned by the steadying symmetry of square grid lines.

Bewildered, he slid the accordion-folded map out of its manila sheath. He had never seen it before. He didn't understand what it was doing in this envelope. The connection of why it was there was still several long moments away.

From the worn interior corners where the color had given way to disintegrating paper stock, he deduced the map had seen countless cycles of use. As he gingerly pulled its folds apart, the legend appeared, spilling part of its mystery.

Don swallowed hard.

"Vietnam, Cambodia, Laos, and Thailand."

He froze for a moment, staring at the colorful depiction of the place he lost himself in so long ago.

The wall map had been produced by the cartographic division of *National Geographic* magazine. It was a supplement to the cover story for the publication's February 1967 Volume 131, No. 2.

Its glossy cover bore the solemn but inviting eyes of a Viet youth whose upward gaze is framed by the traditional conical hat of the country's peasantry. The cover story sought to introduce America to the Vietnam behind the war headlines—a distant country and ancient culture that most Americans knew nothing about.

Don's mind scrolled backwards. His aunt bought him the subscription to *National Geographic* for his eighth birthday, and his family were devoted readers of the publication ever since. For a moment, he lost himself in the innocent boy so many years ago, eyes wide with wonder, thumbing through the brightly colored pages of pictures from distant exotic lands.

He would have received this edition in the mail only months before he graduated high school in June of 1967. Vietnam was still a far-off corner of the world he surely would only see depicted in photographs. He couldn't have known how wrong he was.

Don felt himself reluctantly return to the dimness of his garage. The edges of the map trembled as he held it in front of him.

He cautiously unfolded it like a delicate present he wasn't sure he wanted. However, curiosity drove past his reluctance. He wanted to find his combat area of operations. He needed to see where his little corner of hell fit into the grander scheme of the country that forever changed his life. But more perplexing was the reason the map was tucked into his father's box of treasures.

The looming questions drew him towards the middle panel of the map corresponding to the multicolored elevations of Vietnam's Central Highlands. With a jolt, both questions suddenly answered themselves.

He didn't need to look for names that sounded unintelligible to the tuning of the American ear. He didn't search for the locations that once meant nothing to him, but now filled countless graves in his memory. He didn't need to find the places he had left parts of his soul. The search was unnecessary.

The blue ink was still vibrant considering its age.

Don was transfixed on the irregular swath it cut through the earthy hues depicting the mountains in which the 4th Infantry operated. The stoic blue path felt strange, as if somehow, he was looking at someone else's war. Perhaps this is what it looked like to the generals, he thought.

Suddenly, he felt a sickening wave of vertigo as everything started moving. His mind careened ahead, pulling forth his past. It assembled the chaotic rush of fragmented memories into the coherent sequence following the trail of blue ink. The map came alive, and poured itself all over him.

Before, when the war beckoned him, Don tried the familiar tricks to turn it off. He would have steadied his nerves with a drink. Or three.

This time, Don stood his ground. Without any conscious effort, he felt his emotional core stiffen. As he found traction, the nausea faded, and he found his way back to the present. Remnants of his previous work in therapy clicked into place.

"Hmmm," he thought to himself. "Maybe Doc was right. Dragons only chase you when you run."

He looked down at it again. And as his eyes anchored themselves to the map, he studied the blue lines. His mind shifted to the second, more perplexing question. It was then it struck him.

The effort. The interest. The caring....

The tears came, the thought coming not far behind.

He cared. Dad really cared.

Then another epiphany. Don considered what he worked so hard to learn in his recovery; their relationship lived on within him. Though his father had been dead for years, the map gave them another chance. Another chance to heal a wound he was still carrying. Another chance to forgive.

Don now had a son of military age. He closed his eyes and imagined his son being called up for war. Then the perspective shift came easily.

Fifty-two years earlier, his father set aside the map of Volume 131, No. 2. He combed Don's letters for information. A province. A town. A village. A hill name or number.

He needed something—anything to fill the void left by his son fighting thousands of miles from home. He just needed to know where Don was, even if the fresh blue dot on the map was obsolete by the time the hastily written letters traveled from across the globe. Anything to plug the void of uncertainty.

Standing in his garage, all these years later, Don felt his gut shift. Then an ache he had carried all of his adult life, dissolved. And something long-dislocated finally fell into place.

His father cared.

Don just couldn't let it in at the time. He was running from his own demons. And he hadn't yet become a father, so he couldn't feel the love driving his father's intrusive need to know. But he could now.

It lay in front of him as clearly as the trail of meticulously drawn blue ink. His father never said a word about the map. Now, no words were necessary.

Don took a deep breath and the tears welled up through the depths. Through years of distance and tension. Through years of resentment. The emotion crested, then came to rest.

He smiled as he tucked the map back into the Point Beer crate. Alongside his father's keepsakes, he carefully placed the lightly rusted thirty-round AK magazine, the enameled rice bowl, war pictures, war leaflets and the battle scarred NVA canteen he claimed from the jungle floor.

The remnants of that awful time would now rest together in the faded Point Beer crate.

Complete. And in peace.

22

The Resident

I hadn't taken a psychiatry student in for group therapy training for years. I only agreed to help a psychiatrist colleague out of a bind; he needed to find his resident an elective rotation placement on short notice. I regretted my assent almost as soon as I gave it.

I'd seen too many of them before. Most medical students viewed their psychiatry rotation as a "get through" on their way to their true areas of interest. I began spinning fantasies about how this would go.

My incoming student was a fourth-year medical resident with a name I couldn't pronounce who probably would be wearing a bow tie and unapologetically looking at his watch wondering how quickly he could get out of the room.

The story I told myself was that he would be rolling his eyes when he saw my group leadership model. I started feeling self-conscious about putting my group work on display and wondering how he would judge my craft. My mind narrated the imagined conversation.

"Process therapy? Are there really people still doing that? Are you still using leeches to bleed your patients?"

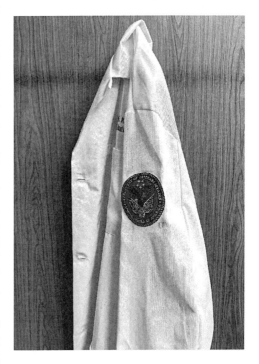

Author's photograph.

I was guarded when I first met him, though was disarmed by his kind, soft eyes. The fantasy I constructed started pulling on that thread fully expecting his veneer to unravel into the truth I had created about him. But that was short-lived.

Those gentle eyes gave way to a curious and surprisingly open intellect. As we talked, I eased my hasty narrative as I collected more information about this stranger in front of me. We discussed issues of contemporary PTSD practice and adjacent psychiatry subjects in which I thought he would take interest. I scanned hard for arrogance and impatience. I found humility and curiosity. He was not who I expected.

The resident didn't know it, but he passed my initial trust screening. I told myself that it was my responsibility to screen him to protect my patients, and that was true. However, the deeper truth was I was also looking to protect myself. The field continued to shift away from my group therapy approach and couldn't wait to catch up to the medical field in wholesale adoption of evidence-based practice. If therapy wasn't written into a protocol, they didn't embrace it anymore. Accordingly, I had become more wary of who I let into the sacred circles of my group therapy patients.

Though this screening went well enough, the real test was waiting on the other side of the door. Traumatized combat veterans are a tough jury. After I provided the doctor some initial group decorum instructions, we walked into the therapy room.

The room was packed—there were twenty-two Vietnam vets with PTSD staring at the new presence among us. We took our seats, and after a pause of awkward silence, I shifted the group into action. The veterans must have judged him as harmless because they immediately took off triaging the order of business. And there was something pressing that day.

Though the veteran's acute crisis had already passed, we began processing his recent psychiatric hospitalization. With anxiety-riddled stuttering and tremulous hands, the just-discharged veteran explained to his peers how he "lost it" in advance of an imminent, but long-feared and avoided, truth-finding mission to the Army National Archives in Washington, D.C.

This veteran put off this pilgrimage for years. He was hoping to find information about his line unit in the 4th Infantry Division, and their combat missions into neutral neighboring countries that were kept from public view during the war. Among his many horrific experiences in Vietnam, this stood out as the worst; he needed to find out why so many of his friends were slaughtered in the winter of 1968. They died on an undocumented, and in the veteran's view, covered-up incursion on an unknown hill somewhere just across the Cambodian/Laotian border.

Before his mental collapse, the veteran was readying himself for this trip to those archives in D.C. to start the excavation process. He wanted to know the truth.

No. *Needed* to know it.

But the pressure of his imminent departure date was too much. The nightmares mounted, his sleep evaporated, and the collision of anxiety and exhaustion became too much. As the veteran shared his humbling decompensation, time melted into the group's process and disappeared. He dug deep and took everyone in the room with him into that abyss. He spoke with vivid detail and within minutes, we found ourselves with him, on that hill, somewhere across the border, aching for the young men who died in that unknown place. The testimony was raw in its power, truth, and emotion. By the group's end, we sat stunned, overcome with empathy, tears flowing freely, and in respectful silence of his story.

The resident followed me to my office for our planned debriefing. I was anxious to ask him about his experience after the intense and dynamic group session. I braced for the anticipated judgments.

"That was … amazing!"

Wrong again. I slowly exhaled.

We discussed why he found it so and I came to see not the arrogant resident-in-training I had initially imagined, but a sensitive, gentle, and eager learner who just had an experience like never before.

The next session he attended was better yet; the group didn't skip a beat and the room filled with emotionally searing truths about combat trauma rarely found outside of these walls. After exiting the group room and making our way to my office, I asked what his reactions were to the session he just witnessed.

He sat staring at me, his lower lip quivering slightly, looking the way my young son did when signaling tears were on the way. And they came.

He offered a raw, heartfelt account of his experience and then connected it to his own traumatic past. In my two decades of supervising psychology doctoral students, I rarely heard someone share so deeply and authentically. Any lingering judgments I harbored disappeared.

"I felt like crying the entire session. I could feel what they were feeling and relate to it. I have never seen or been a part of anything like this in my life."

He explained there was a civil war in his home country of Nepal when he was younger, and hinted at the trauma he experienced there. Though my instinct craved details, he was my student, not my patient, so I simply listened. I intuited from his testimony that he tasted fear and knew human ugliness, and that was enough to earn my respect and his initiation into our sacred circle.

He also shared his struggles in America as an alienated stranger in a foreign land without his family for support. He, too, felt scared and alone just like so many of the veterans in the group that day when they returned "home." He shared the challenges of managing his profound sense of disconnection from this culture so unlike his own, and who judged him just as I had. He held the mirror, and I saw, with a jolt of shame, my shrouded prejudice reflected back.

Never did he believe that he would find a psycho-spiritual kinship with an older generation of American combat veterans whom he had never met, and on the other side of the globe so far from home. Subsequent sessions in the group only deepened this sense of identification and connection. When his final session came, I felt sincere regret at his departure.

"When I came here, I didn't think I would fit in. But I feel just like they do ... what they were describing, their emotions. I didn't think that was possible. I am so grateful for this experience. Thank you so much!"

The resident's energized handshake and effusive smile conveyed genuine gratitude. This affirmed the reason the veterans came back week after week to their group therapy sessions; they were getting what they needed. The resident had no idea what to expect when he arrived, but he also got what he needed. As did I.

I then remembered why I originally loved training. But I had to face my doubts first.

I needed to recall that in recent years, I felt I didn't have as much to offer, that training programs were more interested in protocols than process, and that they valued empirical method over the healing art of being a psychotherapist rooted in philosophy and our shared humanity as much as science. The truth was I increasingly wondered if my art form was passé.

I was telling myself a story that I no longer had something of value to pass on and that training was better left to recently graduated colleagues who had been inculcated with "newer" models. My veterans were teaching me what they needed, while my field and employer waved me in another direction. It's hard to walk your path alone, head and heart conflicted. The challenge was keeping my true north while the compass, according to others, should have read a different azimuth. Professionally, I was struggling through my own dark night of the soul.

However, I know what I see happen when I bring healing to my veterans. I observe their response to my helping them in ways that select few know how to do. I was asking them to find trust in their own healing process. I needed to do the same.

Combat veterans divide their social world into two rather unforgiving categories—you either "get it"...

...or you don't.

So much of a veteran's social pain and alienation comes from being surrounded by those who don't get it. While I continue to learn from the veterans every day, I know I "get it." I only know this because the veterans taught me that I do. But my education of that truth never stops.

The resident reminded me that we are all, at once, teachers and students: I taught him, and he taught me. Just as my veterans continue to do on a daily basis. He reminded me of the lesson that prejudice and judgments obscure our ability to connect with and truly understand one another.

The Nepalese doctor left as quickly as he entered. But he came along just in time, leaving each of us with the parting gift of connection and affirming truths we both needed to remember.

23

Just Shoot Me

Being creatures of habit, it's probably a good thing that we can't foresee life's twists and turns and the changes they demand of us. If we did, we'd likely spend much of our time frozen in fear.

I didn't like the prospect of my right flank in the group circle being exposed by the empty space John's absence would create. His steadfast character and unbroken attendance were as reassuring to me as it was to his Thursday morning PTSD group for many years now. But another change was coming.

John suffered from quadriplegia. His large, motorized wheelchair held his similarly large frame, but his presence went far beyond the physical. The incredible obstacles in his life shaped him into the man that every member of his group grew to respect. We witnessed him face and conquer many such challenges.

But the surgery next week was different; it would be preparing him for the start of dialysis and the time-consuming filtering process that would help prevent his single failing kidney from killing him.

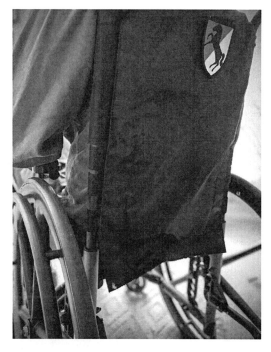

Author's photograph.

"I'm not looking forward to this, but I don't have a choice. The doctor said my remaining kidney is functioning at eleven percent. After that last surgery, he said with some surprise that he wasn't sure he would ever see me again, so nothing is guaranteed. They are trying to set it up so I can do the dialysis at home, but I'm not sure what this may mean for my schedule. I hope to be able to come back to the group but we will have to see how this goes," John explained to the concerned ring of twelve fellow Vietnam combat veterans.

Having a spinal cord injury involved much in the way of time and effort that most cannot fathom. John required the help of a full-time assistant to get him out of bed and two hours to prepare him for each day. His bedtime routine was no picnic either. He spent many hours of his day doing what most people encounter as trivial inconveniences. He now had to bear the additional burden of several hours of dialysis. It dawned on us that this life-saving commitment was the end his group membership.

At first, the other veterans rushed to support him in facing yet another surgery—he had endured too many. And the chain reaction of problems had all started with Vietnam. Agent orange poisoned his body and he suffered from multiple systemic illnesses that government acknowledgment eventually tied to the defoliant used heavily in his area of operations. However, it was decades before he would learn that this legacy of the war laid hidden in his body. He left Vietnam alive, but harboring the toxic seeds of what was to come.

John was initially ambivalent about joining the Army. However, he had a military tradition in his family and, to him, it was simply the right thing to do. While he volunteered for service, he attributed his eventual drive to excel to a drill instructor who noticed John's hesitancy and pulled him aside during basic training to adjust his attitude.

"It's time you stop asking what the Army can get out of you and time to ask what you can get out of the Army," the Sergeant both suggested and commanded.

This was as close to a good piece of advice one could hope for from a DI and John dutifully absorbed the instruction. He graduated first in his class from boot camp and went on to NCO school before shipping to Vietnam where he served as a Sergeant with the 11th Armored Cavalry. Their mechanized infantry unit operated in the VC-infested 3rd Corps war zone east of Saigon.

As the punishing sun faded on yet another day of patrol in the field, his unit arranged their armored personnel carriers in a night defensive position and began to dig in. John warily surveyed the darkening wood line just in front of their circled vehicles.

Even with their .50 caliber machine guns bristling outward like fearsome metal quills, he didn't like the looks of this. Had it been his decision, he would have set up further away from the jungle's dense, ominous edge.

The enemy were just too good at using the terrain to compensate for their inferior firepower. To fight the Americans, they had to do more with less. They learned to "grab by the belt"—the Vietnamese military doctrine of pulling in so close to fight their American enemy that it neutralized the primary advantages of devastating air and artillery power. In a toe-to-toe fight, their ill-equipped guerrilla force was no match.

That's why the enemy rarely squared off in a pitched battle, and their tactics constantly mutated. When a vulnerability appeared, somehow the VC appeared to exploit it before melting back into the jungle like phantoms.

John's unit learned many of these lessons the hard way. John didn't like the look of this place. But it wasn't his call. The cover of darkness came fast.

From the tree line, a rocket-propelled grenade with its glowing vapor trail shrieked towards his APC. The explosion showered its occupants with molten shrapnel.

Before John knew what was happening, he lay wounded and blinded while the subsequent attack raged around him. The fight lasted hours. The best his besieged men could do was shelter him behind his track while he lay helpless in muffled darkness, the bloodied compression bandages encircling his head. It was the last night John would ever see out of his left eye again.

While that was the end of his war, it was hardly John's last battle. The surgeons were unable to save his eye. Some years later, this partial blindness resulted in an industrial accident which broke his neck. The damage to his spinal cord was considered an "incomplete" cervical injury and, in that moment, he became a quadriplegic and confined to a wheelchair for the rest of his life.

Though the VA hospital had a state-of-the-art spinal cord injury unit, he was told that the life expectancy of a man with his injuries was likely ten to fifteen years. Odds were slim John would see fifty years of age.

But he was a survivor in every sense of the word. In spite of this dire prognosis, he went on to live a full and productive life. He enjoyed a career, got married, had a family, and was involved in his church. As if he hadn't suffered enough, one day he received a call that his wife was killed in a car accident. He eventually recovered from this devastating loss, remarried, and moved on as he had so many times before.

In spite of his nonnegotiable dependence on others, John's independence, wherever possible, was likewise, non-negotiable. His van was fitted with custom controls and a lift to allow him the freedom of the road. Aside from his obvious disabilities, no one would have suspected that the mental trauma of the war lay dormant within him. In fact, to hear him tell his story, it wasn't until his body became wracked with various illnesses tied to his agent orange exposure that the ghosts of Vietnam intruded back into his life.

When it did, a slumbering anger awoke, often triggered by frustrations he experienced as a disabled man in an able-bodied world. On many occasions, these two worlds collided.

Though no longer in much of a position to fight, John was not one to retreat. Especially from someone who required a courtesy lesson. He was shocked by the number of other people that valued a closer parking spot over respect for others who truly needed them. And he lost count of the times others ignored the signs designed to clear the adjacent space for his van's lift.

On one such occasion, a particularly obstinate offender required some additional training in civility. After a brief exchange, he wound up facing the business end of John's .45 pistol. This didn't legally end well for either of them, but was instrumental in convincing both John and his increasingly concerned family that he needed some help.

In spite of John's need to spend incalculable amounts of time at medical appointments, he had never darkened the door of a mental health professional before. One therapist in our PTSD program suggested group therapy and, though he was reluctant, John figured he would see what he could get out of it. Like boot camp, it worked for him once before.

He sat silently for a few group sessions and just listened. He witnessed other veterans in the group discuss, with shocking transparency, their many struggles with the war and the ways it had impacted them. Then came the revelation.

"Holy shit. You guys are talking about me!"

John found his struggling warrior image reflected in the mirror. This group of men whose lives were fundamentally altered by the war didn't care to cut the corners of polite social discourse. John listened. Men were speaking the truth. Then, one day, John gambled on speaking his own.

The group listened to his story without judgment and offered their reactions. They validated his experience. And they validated *him*—assuring that his struggles were welcomed here. No longer did his war have to hide. John finally opened the door to the journey back home.

That was many years ago and after realizing he had much to learn in this group of men, he continued to attend virtually every week. In spite of his challenges, he kept coming. While it happened gradually, his anger melted away.

The group cherished what was left in its wake. His love, humor, and thoughtfulness shone through his comments to others and when he had something to work on, we all looked for the precious and unhurried lesson that was coming. We had much to learn from the man who had overcome his countless daily struggles with a buoyant demeanor that we could only marvel at. His slow Tennessean, southern drawl only added to his enviable tranquility and the lingering grip of his narrative.

He became more open at home and his family supported his treatment. John recounted a conversation with his brother, who had been rather skeptical of his allegiance to this weekly gathering of aging warriors. His brother cynically asked, "Does that group *really* do you any good?"

John thought for a moment, smiled, and replied in his leisurely southern cadence.

"Well.... Let's see.... I haven't pulled a gun on anyone in over six years. I would have to say it does." His smile broadened, dually signaling the pride in the accomplishment and the amusement of using such a metric to measure his recovery progress.

His brother was speechless. It was hard to argue with a result like that.

It was in this potentially last therapy session of his that John recounted this interaction with his brother again. The group didn't mind that he had told that story several times before. His fresh delivery brought the same laughs from men who didn't find the solution of pulling guns on others when necessary as absurd at all. While they applauded his growth, his six year "abstinence" was also part of the joke.

Once you shed the oft-naive civilian mindset constructed upon a safe world without regular threat of violent attack or the necessity of being armed to fight it, one came to appreciate the naked humor of men who had been to war. But today, the story didn't feel as funny. It had the mournful edge of a goodbye. In what had been a lifetime full of them, this wasn't just going to be another surgery.

It was the jarring realization that the group might lose this anchor of a man. A man who taught the group they were capable of overcoming anything life would throw in their path—a path we silently pleaded wouldn't change but then suddenly vanished, only to open another uncertainty before us. His life had seen so many of these shifts, and he managed to find meaning in them all.

That's why one veteran needed an answer. *His* answer.

"John—I just don't think I could go through it. Everything you've been through. I just don't think I could...."

"Well, Len ... had I known what I would have to go through to get where I am today ... well.... I would've said, 'just shoot me.'"

Though no one said so, the group's quiet energy suggested a collective sigh of relief. It was the comforting realization that this man was no different than any other man in the room. His resilience came from a very mortal place. It made John's enviable peace feel attainable to us all.

The relief penetrated deeper layers. If we were willing to be honest, in the face of such catastrophic hurdles, shooting oneself might have even seemed rational. The relief then gave way to inspiration. It reminded the group that, like us all, John was just another human being whose fate was better left unknown. Because he didn't know how high the mountain was, he took it one plateau at a time, learning the critical lessons as he went.

But he kept going.

That day in the group, these veterans shared a thoughtful dialogue about the role of perspective, resilience, and taking the challenges as they come. We explored their reflections on their lives, and their self-assessments of what they could handle and what they feared they could not. Many lost sight of their own strengths in the glare of John's. It was now his turn to hold the mirror so the group could see their own triumphs over tragedy.

The blinding irony was striking given their collective patchwork of physical and emotional stories of resilience: they had all survived a war that over 58,000 didn't. Many were severely wounded in combat and bore the Purple Hearts to prove it. Many faced social ostracism and rejection by the very public in whose name they went to war. And that was just their "homecoming."

After returning from overseas, one group member went back to the same tough city streets he was raised in. He became hooked on heroin, and while he didn't get a scratch in Vietnam, he would take a shotgun blast to the abdomen some years later. He had since gotten clean, and was no longer caught in the cycle of drugs and violence. He was one of the stronger and more fortunate ones. As he now reflects, many he used to run with on those streets weren't so lucky.

Another group member struggling with his then-untreated PTSD symptoms lost his job, his income, and his home. He lived in his car for as long as he could. When that became untenable, he retreated to the tunnels under the city streets where he joined a community of homeless subterranean dwellers. He survived in this makeshift underground camp until he got his disability benefits and a way out of the darkness.

John was one of four men who had survived early tragic deaths of their spouses. One group member, a former city EMT, only narrowly missed the call that would have unexpectedly brought him to the scene of a multi-casualty motor vehicle accident where, upon the bloodied asphalt, his own wife lay among the dead.

Another veteran lost the love of his life to an early cancer death only to meet a second true love who just recently succumbed to the same fate. He had only just recovered from a severe depression that he hoped would take him down far enough to end his pain. However, he fought his way out of that depressive episode and was in the early stages of contemplating a reinvention of himself. Another group member and former maximum-security prison guard survived a lethal shank attack by two inmates which left him stabbed multiple times while his partner lay dead on the floor. Several in the group survived their children. The group's roster of triumph over tragedy didn't stop there—it went on and on.

However, especially today, all eyes were on John. They needed to touch the perseverance and hope he embodied. They needed to tap his spirit and catch its reflected light back to them. They needed to let him know how much they cared about him and would miss him should he not be able to make his way back to them.

And they needed to be prepared to say goodbye.

One of the men going through his own dark transition addressed him.

"John—you have been through so much, suffered more than any one of us, and yet you are the happiest man in this room. I need you here. We love you. I love you."

That day, we watched the happiest man in the room smile, shake hands with his friends and fellow elder warriors, accept their well wishes, and drive his wheelchair out through the door into the next unknown.

⁓

Epilogue: This story was completed a few months before John eventually went on dialysis. He continued to suffer from one medical crisis after the next and was in and out of the hospital for several months. During one of these multiple admissions, he contracted COVID-19. The last time we saw him (in a virtual group session), he was as positive as ever, though was noticing the onset of cold symptoms. Just before Veterans Day in the fall of 2020, he entered the hospital for the last time before succumbing to the virus.

24

The Adopted

Mark cleared his throat to start off the group therapy session, but the tears started flowing before he could finish his first sentence. Hearing this cue, the Friday morning PTSD group came to order. The room fell silent to clear the path for whatever was coming.

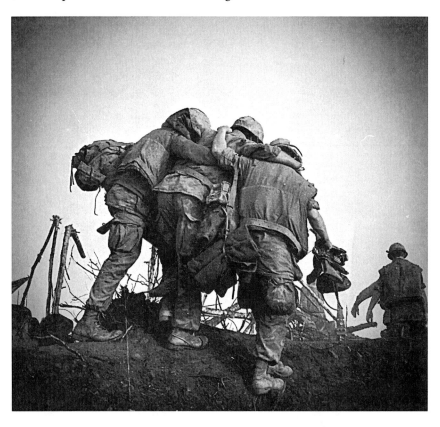

Marine helped to evacuation point, National Archives, photograph 532463.

To a man, these Vietnam combat veterans struggled with the holidays for so many reasons. Thanksgiving had just passed and Christmas was coming fast. Mark prepared to update the group on the family Thanksgiving he discussed with anxious anticipation the previous group session.

He always struggled with how to "be" during holidays, mostly because of the list of hidden expectations attached to them. He wasn't much for small talk. He couldn't feel the pleasure he saw others wearing and the careless ease with which they flowed through the maze of people, oblivious to his plight. Though surrounded by others, he felt so utterly alone.

And they reminded him of what he lost somewhere in the jungle. Mark couldn't remember the last time he enjoyed what he saw in their festive expressions. His head was filled with too much—too much anger. Too much despair. Too much fear.

The holidays were hard enough. But this one was worse.

This Thanksgiving dinner invitation came with the promise of a surprise.

Mark didn't like surprises. Surprises may have added to the fun for others. But not for him.

Ever since Vietnam, he had too many fears to dump into the void of anything he couldn't see coming. Bracing for whatever horror he imagined just around that blind corner was so deeply ingrained. It kept him alive over there but refused to leave after he came home. The fear sat vigil over his every move, his every thought, his every feeling. If anyone picked up on the tension, a hollow offering usually followed. "That was a long time ago," they would assure him. "You're home now."

They didn't get it. How could they? They weren't there.

The entire war was built on the rickety scaffolding of the fear of the uncertain. The dread would set in while saddling up for a mission before being delivered into the jaws of the unknown. And if you survived that one, there was another mission waiting right behind it. When that day was done, night would come. A grunt would pray to see the morning sun. If it came up for him that first day, he had 364 and a wake-up to go until he could leave this place. Most learned to stop counting.

Mark served with the 9th Infantry Division in the Mê Kông Delta near Đồng Tâm. He spent the first part of his tour with the grunts and later trained as a sniper. He earned two air medals and almost secured a third, each representing twenty-five combat air assaults. He was choppered into too many LZs where the unknown sickened him with impending doom. He always felt fear on the way in, and the short-lived ecstasy of survival on the way out. It was the between part that haunted him.

Once on foot, the ominous wood lines whose impenetrable wall of brush often hid a camouflaged enemy until it was too late. The eerie still-ness would suddenly explode around him. A man's nerves rarely had a chance to recover. In Vietnam, the pucker factor just stayed too high, too long.

So, during the war Mark learned to dread surprises for the simple rea-son that he lived in perpetual fear of attack. He never knew when it was coming. A lot of times the attack never came. Too many times it did. Soon, it became hard to tell one from the other.

Mark told the group how he braced for the worst while anticipating the Thanksgiving family gathering. As it neared, he battled alternating waves of anxiety and depression. To make matters worse, he ran out of his antidepressant meds which typically broke his fall.

But by now, he made it through Thanksgiving Day surprise already. The calendar was now rounding December. On his trauma recovery jour-ney, he had cried so many times because of the fear and pain. But this time, his tears were those of relief, of gratitude, and … of joy.

"I'm going to be a grandfather!" he announced with a gleaming smile framed by tears running down both cheeks.

Then he narrated his Thanksgiving Day surprise for us.

He heard the muffled clamor of familiar voices in conversation as he hesitantly made his way up the paved walkway. The cool fall air padded the beads of sweat on his forehead. He paused at the front door and took a moment to work up the nerve to walk through his dread and into the house.

The aromas of Thanksgiving dinner were the first to greet him. He quickly scanned the room looking for something to stuff into the gaping void. The fear evaporated the instant he saw her.

It was his oldest daughter, the one previously thought unable to con-ceive. He was greeted by her rotund belly and a glowing smile that melted his heart.

The dilemma set in later. His joy felt foreign—dangerous even.

Joy was a luxury a man constantly scanning for the next threat could ill afford. Something deep within him began calculating the risks of what he couldn't yet see—the opaque fate of his daughter and unborn grand-child. Nine months was a big unknown. Too much time for something to go wrong. Since Vietnam, he always feared punishment for his actions during the war.

And it wasn't just Mark. Many of the veteran's surrounding him struggled with that same conviction. Mark worked hard in his therapy to free himself, but his guilt patiently shadowed him at every turn. There were too many times in combat he wished he could change, but couldn't. Some hurt worse than others.

Mark reminded the group which memory now threatened to take his joy away. He discussed this trauma in this group before so it required only two words to reconnect us to the story that refused to leave him in peace.

It was the *old man.*

He probably was a grandfather too. Now that Mark was about to become one, he confessed his haunting new fear to the group.

Would his past errors during the war bring God's wrath upon his unborn grandchild? Would the child or his daughter's health suffer because Mark had caused others to suffer? Would he have to feel the karmic pain of the same loss the old man's family felt when he never returned home to his village?

The old man didn't come home that day because he had fallen to a sniper's bullet.

Mark's bullet. Of the countless rounds he had fired during the war, it was the one he wished he could take back.

In his therapy, Mark left no stone unturned. He examined that mission in every detail—the tactical situation, the chain of events set in motion that were beyond his control, and the split-second, instinctive decision to act in the heat of the moment that changed his life forever. He could hear the echoes of his shouting "No!" as one of the riflemen on his flank mistakenly triggered the ambush. There were no armed VC in the kill zone.

Just an old man and a boy.

Mark came to accept that much of the situation was beyond him, but in the end, he couldn't change one painful fact—he pulled the trigger.

Mark was forever tethered to the life he took that day. The old man visited him in his nightmares, his blood-covered face looking up at him as Mark stood overly the mortally wounded village elder lying on the trail. He would awaken with a start, smothered in sweat and despair.

In therapy, Mark struggled to come to uneasy terms with this soul wound. He fought to reconcile that young sniper and the man he was now. Though early in the process, he slowly accepted the man he became; a deeply sensitive, caring man with love in his heart. A man deserving of compassion for the soldier who did the best he could in the disorienting vortex of war. And, in his view, a man destined to carry the burden for two souls for the rest of his life.

Mark searched for the path that might lead him to trust himself again. To trust the truth of who he was. And the grandfather he would become.

The group rallied around him. They challenged the aging fears that threatened to undermine it. They celebrated his joy and fought to allow him to keep it. They tied this to the running theme of our work focused on exploring the risks of change—of rewriting well-worn pathways of expectation, of self-condemnation, and fear of the "what if's."

They were exploring moving beyond being defined by their trauma to become the men they wished to be. Needed to be. Deserved to be.

Mark exhaled deeply, and smiled as he finished his work for the day. However, as was common during the group process, there were an infinite number of ways our work activated hidden pockets of pain. As Mark thanked the group for providing the safe space share his joy and fears, hurt had found another man in the room.

Joseph's face was red with anguish and tears were starting to flow. Though unintended, Mark's joy reflected Joseph's greatest pain.

"I'm the only man in this room who didn't have children of my own. And when I'm dying, I'm not going to have my son or daughter by my bedside. I'm going to die alone," Joseph said.

The gravity of that image sank in before he continued.

"I read my bible, and I wonder if I was destined to be cursed … denied the sacred gift of children because of the things I've done."

Joseph had other regrets, but the pain of being childless was perhaps his biggest. Soon after returning from Vietnam, he married. His first wife didn't want children and by the time their unhappy union of thirty-three years ended in divorce, it was too late—his window for fatherhood had passed. His pain poured into the room and, once again, the room rallied.

Though he hadn't fathered his own, he was not without children in his life. In fact, he had more young souls move through his life than he could count.

After the war, Joseph attended college and then earned two master's degrees in psychology and physical education. He taught in high school and became a PE coach.

At first, he tried applying the same respect-commanding skills to his students as he had as an Army Ranger Sergeant in Vietnam. However, as the bottomless needs of so many of his students rushed at him, the learning began to flow in both directions. And Joseph began to change.

He learned to earn their respect rather than command it. Toughness and orders gave way to kindness and listening. He provided them time, attention, and an open mind. He built them up instead of tearing them down. He offered what he never had as a child and so many of them were missing.

And the children loved him for it.

Yes, Joseph never raised his own children, but the number he fathered in deeds and spirit was countless.

The group brilliantly supported him. They gave him the space for his sadness while reminding him of the number of children still carrying the impact of his loving attention long after his retirement.

The sadness clung to him, but he was beginning to feel the truth he was hearing. Then he told the story of the girl with an absent father who came to him in great need. He talked to her and offered her his phone number if she ever needed to talk. She never took him up on that call.

Many years later a woman he didn't recognize approached him in a store. The years had changed her appearance, but when he heard her voice, he knew. Had she not said anything, her smile and grateful eyes might have said it all.

But she did say something. She thanked him for being there for her when her father wasn't. That call never came because he already gave her a gift—a man who didn't need the title of father just to care like one.

And there were many others, such as the thin girl in tattered hand-me-downs who, upon seeing him, would wrap herself around him like a koala bear. Like many kids in Joseph's classes, she didn't have a father at home who saw what his daughter needed. Mirroring her slight frame, emotionally she was starving. Though Joseph appreciated her honest affection and granting of trust, he set the limits with her in a loving way, taking great care not to reject her feelings.

The truth was that he deeply valued providing other kids with the love and attention he had longed for, but did not receive, as a child. He knew that in today's world, the rules were there for good reason; it wouldn't have taken much for an on-looker to get the wrong idea about something so innocently right.

There were many more stories he shared that the group reminded him should be added to that list. They celebrated the ways he was a father figure to so many school children who needed one so badly. Kids that knew he cared.

The healing energy in the group that day expanded to envelop both Mark and Joseph. Yet another man could have fallen into his own old wounds, but Gene took another direction. He also happened to be sitting right beside Joseph.

These were two large men—big in physical stature, intellect, and spirit. They also shared a kinship as their tours in Vietnam were in close parallel; they both served in elite recon units and were bonded by the small-team guerrilla combat they survived.

Gene, a mountain of a man, turned to Joseph, tenderly looked at his brother in arms and starkly explained the bottom line of his childhood:

"I was adopted. My mother gave me up because I was too much of a bother. They had trouble finding a family for me because I was so big. That's not guessing. I've done the research. I was supposed to go to a good, religious Catholic home. Only that didn't happen. My father brought his own unhealed PTSD back from WWII. He beat me regularly, and my mother didn't do much to stop it. I got no love there. So, I had a father but never really had a dad."

Joseph nodded—he knew that pain. Tears streamed down his face before disappearing into his trimmed platinum and gray mustache. Gene shifted in his chair to look him in the eye to make sure he knew that what came next was for real.

"So now I'm adopting you. You're my dad. You're the father I wished I would have had."

Gene smiled at his newly adoptive father. Eyes red and swollen with tears, Joseph smiled back. These two elder warriors, now in their 70s, sat astride as a newly minted "family of choice."

The room chuckled at the playful declaration. In exploring the sacred gift of children and grandchildren and the pain of absent fathers, they found another embedded reward—the healing borne of their living brotherhood. Children were a sacred gift. But so were these connections in the group. As combat veterans attest, they are deeper than family.

Though oblivious to the passing of time, the clock struck noon in the next moments signaling the end of the session.

Exchanging silent smiles, handshakes, hugs and whispered gratitude, the band of elder warriors slowly filed out of the room, lingering a moment or two longer in the room's radiance before venturing back outside.

25

Buddha's Treasure

Peter gripped the knotted sandwich baggie in his hand. He asked for the opportunity to start the session of our Tuesday afternoon PTSD group. I nodded before he requested that we each draw one from the bag before passing it to the man to his left.

In the bag was an assortment of patinaed coins. Their distinctive features reflected the troubled history of Vietnam. The currencies traced the foreign empires who occupied the country only to eventually be ejected before another took its place. Some were stamped with Chinese characters, others from the French Colonial period, and several with a hole through the center reflecting antiquity's practice of wearing one's wealth.

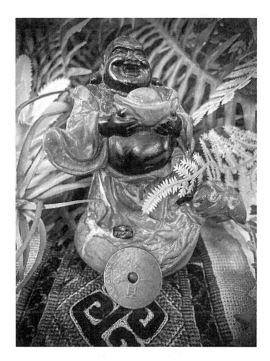

Author's photograph.

With great reverence, every group member selected the coin which felt right to them, and passed the bagged jumble around the circle of ten men. As they did so, Peter narrated the story of how he came to possess this treasure.

In 1967, his unit, Kilo Company, 3rd Battalion, 1st Marines, was on a sweep mission in I Corps when his fireteam came upon a bombed-out church. The structure was odd for a number of reasons. It had been constructed of brick, a rare building material in their area of operations, and stood conspicuously isolated in the otherwise desolate and raw war-torn landscape.

The Marines scouted the ruins. Peter described the blown-out windows and doors, the collapsed walls and the remnants of what used to be its roof timbers chaotically littering the floor like giant pick-up sticks. In the rubble, one of them came across a clay statue of Buddha on an altar which, amazingly, given its fragility relative to the decimated edifice that housed it, was the only object left unscathed.

The Marine removed it from its perch. Its heft was promising. When shook, he smiled at the unmistakable metallic jingle. He irreverently threw the statue against a segment of intact brick wall and, upon shattering, revealed the hidden, glittering treasure trove as it spilled onto the ground.

The fireteam assembled around their good fortune and sorted through the coins. Then, like they shared everything else, equitably divided them among themselves. Upon completion, each Marine had a large handful of this unexpected booty.

The veteran continued to narrate the story to the group of men transfixed by the coin they now held in their hands.

"That was a good day. No one got hurt or killed … and we found something in that war that we believed might be worth something. I wanted a trophy to bring home. I stashed mine when we got back to battalion. The rest of the guys ditched their coins in the field."

Peter explained the stark calculus of that decision.

"They were too heavy. We had to carry everything on our backs and there was no room to hump anything that didn't serve the ultimate purpose of staying alive and fighting the enemy. Food and ammo were just more important."

But for him, bringing something home was important and because of that, he carried his coins in a rucksack through the jungles of Vietnam, came 8,500 miles home, and stowed them for safekeeping for the last fifty years.

I turned towards Peter.

"Why now? You've held on to these coins for all of this time. Why do you gift them to the group now?"

The veteran paused before responding, his tone somber.

"For the last several sessions, we have talked about what's important to us, what we brought back from the war, and the stories behind them. We also talked about who in our worlds care about these things that mean so much to us."

Before Peter continued, a sullen silence filled the room.

"I have three friends. Larry, as we all know, just died. I have another friend. He was a Marine RTO at the Battle of Huế. He was just given six months left to live—cancer. I have one other friend who was just diagnosed with a terminal muscle disease that I don't even know the name of."

Gravity pulled many eyes to the floor as that sunk in.

"So, I've been thinking … who would inherit my things and my stories? I've given some of those coins to one of my grandsons. He's about the only one who ever showed any interest in what I did during the war, but even that is limited and … well … there is no one else. No one else would care. No one but you guys."

There was neither a single man in the room who did not take a coin nor one who was not visibly moved by the now-clear meaning of the gift.

As we held the coins in hand, the group went on. The content shifted from heavy to light, from intimacy towards the conversational.

They reflected on living on C-rations in the field—the individual combat meals that had been packaged in OD steel cans during World War II with the date stamp to prove it. They talked of the times they went without any food or water, sometimes for days, such that the age of their food no longer mattered. They were glad to eat anything.

Well, almost anything. They laughed over the new guys in the outfit who eagerly accepted the near-universally despised meal of ham and motherfuckers out of the C-rations crate.

Excitement mounted over the rare occurrences when they were lucky enough to draw the most valued meal components from the resupply crates. That vote was unanimous, and unquestionably nominated the peaches in sweet syrup. One veteran explained the strategy for humping those peaches in their ruck while awaiting the appearance of the small tin of pound cake. When combined, they created a treat so delicious that it made the war, if only for a few minutes, seem just a little further away. So cherished were peaches and pound cake that this dessert became our group's annual tradition to celebrate the winter holidays.

They talked of other simple warzone pleasures wherever they could be found. They connected and laughed over a shared experience of the small joys and comical situations that could be found even in midst of profound misery, death, and destruction.

One of the combat medics then turned to group leadership to narrate what was happening in the room.

"You see … this is why I can relate with another Vietnam combat veteran without even needing to say anything. All that we shared together over there. You just know…."

He described the ability to look at another veteran's face and sense the intuitive connection reflected in the eyes of the other—a portrait of unique suffering that they shared fifty years ago in the jungles of Vietnam that bonded those who would otherwise be mere strangers.

And now, as they approach the twilight of their lives, struggling to make sense of those experiences, and a way out of their emotional isolation, they come together, every Tuesday, to sit in this circle of brothers—men who know one another's burden, sacrifice and pain without having to ask or be told.

However, on this particular Tuesday, a veteran brought in his coveted treasure discovered a half-century ago in the ashes of war. He told the story of the young Marine who searched for something to bring home from Vietnam for reasons he could not appreciate at the time. In 1967, after surviving thirteen months of combat, he brought home his trophy coins while unaware of the real gift that would take many years of suffering and struggle to unfold—the gift of being "awake." While serving in Vietnam, the young Marine was unaware that Buddha meant "the awakened one." Had he known at the time, he wouldn't have cared. But he was no longer the same person.

It took decades of quest for Peter to heal and become a better, fulfilled and more authentic man. He worked hard for years in treatment to painstakingly piece together the puzzle of his tour in Vietnam, to process his rage, grief, and fear, to resolve his alcoholism, and to mend his broken family. While on this path, he discovered his archetypal elder warrior in the twilight of his journey and, along the way, greatly contributed to the growth and trauma recovery of so many of his fellow veterans.

That day in group, Peter discovered why he has carried his coins all of these years. It was to share his gift—the gift of his story, the gift of his wisdom, and the gift of becoming awake.

It was to share Buddha's treasure.

26

Mrs. Schafer's Requiem

This PTSD group started out as most others did—with an utterly blank canvas. There were infinite possibilities that lay before us, and eighteen men that day sat in the quiet contemplation of that vast potential before the first veteran spoke.

Gene prefaced his coming point by providing some history.

His father, a traumatized World War II combat veteran and POW, took out his own pain and rage on his son with frequent beatings. The internal pressures steadily built, fueling the search for a release of his torment. As with many kids from such situations, this came out in the place offering the greatest relative safety—school.

At the point he was spending more time in trouble than in class, the principal summoned his parents for a meeting—he was out of chances. Upon reflection, Gene was certain the primary reason his family moved to a neighboring town was to change schools. In that era, behaviorally disordered kids weren't seen as suffering so much as they were simply an inconvenient and intolerable management problem.

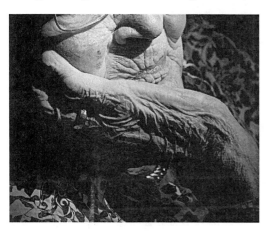

Thus, what the beatings and daily visits to the schoolmaster couldn't correct, a move to another town had to. Upon arriving at his new grade school, he quickly found their schoolyard game of bombardment offered the perfect opportunity.

"It gave me a chance

Geralt, https://pixabay.com/en/woman-old-age-retirement-home-65675.

to discharge my anger—everything I had to carry around with me from those beatings I could take out on someone else and didn't get into trouble for it," Gene introspected to the group.

Absent any social connections, the anonymous players opposing him made tantalizing targets. The new kid wasted little time in attracting the ire of supervising adults on the playground. Gene's conspicuous vigor caught the eye of his classmate's mother, Mrs. Schafer. However, she saw past his unruliness; she saw *him* and something yet unappreciated, but special.

With her character's introduction into the story, the veteran closed the freshly painted portrait he just created for us. The central subject of the scene was the kind attention and compassion Mrs. Schafer extended, and the birth of their special and enduring connection.

Gene turned solemn. It was precisely the special nature of the relationship that set up his current dilemma.

"I think she saved me in many ways, and the reason I'm telling you this now is because Mrs. Schafer just turned ninety-eight and right after her birthday, she had a stroke and ... well ... she doesn't have much time left."

The sadness began to well up in the veteran as he contemplated the near-end of this beautiful soul who looked beyond his behavior, read his suffering, and reached out to him when no one else would. A single tear left its reflective trail as the gravity of his pain pulled it down his cheek.

"My issue is that she's in the hospital and I'm not sure if I can go there and tell her just how much she ... she means to me."

However, his ambivalence with love and connection went even deeper than was immediately apparent. It was digging into another wound.

After Vietnam, Gene worked hard to stay busy and, in so doing, strove to stay one step ahead of the demons from his past. Raising cattle on his rural property was part of that plan. After seeing so much death, he was driven to fill the world with new life. Most of the time, nature took care of that itself. But sometimes, it didn't.

One of Gene's new calves was abandoned by its mother. He became its surrogate; he bottle-fed, nurtured, and raised this lonely calf with loving attention. Their bond deepened and resonated with painful echoes from his own lonely childhood. Gene became the doting parent he never had. The calf later developed pneumonia and, after a mighty struggle to save it, died in his arms. Gene promptly went inside his home, got drunk and attempted to kill himself.

History didn't repeat itself, but sometimes it rhymed. The calf's death cracked open Gene's past and drowned him in an epic flood of memories of his horrific combat tour with the 173rd Airborne in Vietnam.

This backdrop helped the group understand Gene's pain around death and loss. It did not, however, alter the group's consensus about how to handle his dilemma with Mrs. Schafer; death was one thing, but love was a different matter. The verdict was swift and unambiguous—tell her now before it's too late.

The urgent conclusion came from the collective anguish of so many missed opportunities in the room and the incalculable price many paid for that wisdom.

After the war, how many of these men never heard "I love you?" How many saw the true measure of their caring through the opaque layers of emotional callous they had built to protect themselves? Protect themselves from the pain they had carried since their return from Vietnam and, for many, long before that? How many chances had they already squandered? How many did they have left?

As the group reflected on the weight of those costs, some silently began to gravitate back to those familiar dark corners … how many wounded and dead brothers did they put on the medevacs and missed that precious moment to let them know? How many names on the Wall never knew how I loved them….

…how many?

Talking about love in a room filled with hardened combat veterans didn't come easy. But it was too important not to talk about. Eyes shifted to the floor as the silence grew. Legs began bouncing, hoping for some relief, or perhaps courage. The subject refused to leave, so the room sat in its solemn, awkward glow.

Sensing an opening, a lone voice came from across the room.

"Nineteen years ago, I cheated on my wife," started the veteran sitting at the far end of the room. All heads swiveled towards him.

"It wasn't even close to worth it and I ended up hurting the person I loved most in the world." He went on to share how the pain he caused woke him to his self-absorption, his emotional walls, the ways he needed to learn the meaning of love, and how far he has come since.

"For years, I kept telling her how much I love her and she couldn't bring herself to say it—it hurt too bad. I learned my lesson but it came at great cost." I wasn't sure if she would ever forgive me. Then, one day … about five years later, before I left for work, I told her I loved her. And I meant it. And that day, she turned to me and said, 'I love you, too.'"

Silence.

The veteran who shared this had tears running down his cheeks and into the forest of his white, sprawling beard. He then continued.

"My twenty-year-old son just left on a road trip for a concert the other day. I couldn't bear the thought that if something happened to either of us while he was gone, that he wouldn't have heard that from me. That I love him. There were so many during the war I never got to tell them that. They were killed, put in a bag, and then they were gone forever. Now, I tell everyone I love them … and I mean it."

Words scarcely captured the complexity of what happened in a mere ninety minutes. We were all transfixed by what we were creating and the tether of time fell away without any of us noticing. Men spoke of their gratitude for having shared their loving truths with important others before it was too late. Others shared their pain of missing their chance. Broken Relationships. Schisms. Divorces. Deaths.

Others pondered the possibilities laid before them and who in their lives needed to hear their now-opened hearts. Their pain didn't disappear so much as it was enveloped—wrapped in a quilt of connection and rare intimacy woven by this group of warriors. The silent pause that came minutes before session's end signaled our final moments in this healing place.

I don't believe any of us wanted to leave this sanctuary. The sense of connection and naked honesty hung in the air. They felt bonded. They felt understood. And they didn't just understand the love that so many struggled to rediscover after the war that day—they lived it. Like the singular uniqueness of a snowflake, there would never be another group session exactly like it. There was a palpable unspoken appreciation for its preciousness.

I cannot recall a single word I said in my closing remarks. I only know that it sounded as perfect a synthesis as an imperfect artist could construct. I could not think of a more fitting final tribute to the special woman who found the wounded little boy in the school yard that day so many years ago, and extended the love and caring he so thirsted for.

The following week, Gene was not in group. Concerned, several asked if he was okay following last group's intense session. One group member updated the rest of us.

"After last week, some of us were going out to lunch. We asked Gene if he wanted to join us, but he turned down the invitation. He said he had somewhere to go."

Gene went straight to the hospital to see Mrs. Schafer. He got there in time. He told her he loved her.

Two days later, she died.

27

The Crucifix

Clutching the empty space around his neck where it hung for fifty-one years, Don felt a wave of nausea wash over him. He scanned the parking lot beneath him but it was nowhere to be found. The sickening blight of hopelessness brought on by its absence continued to spread. He had been running errands all that morning. It could be anywhere.

When he got home from the store, he retraced his every move while he got ready that morning. He tore apart his dresser drawer where he stowed his keepsakes. He poured through the other tokens from his Vietnam service—there were the propaganda leaflets both sides would litter over the jungle floor, attempting to play on the minds of the battle weary and homesick. There was a small pile of flechettes—the tiny steel darts capable of wicked destruction against soft targets. There were some stained Vietnamese piasters and the presentation boxes cradling his combat service medals and ribbons.

But the crucifix was nowhere.

This wasn't just any crucifix. Don wore it in the jungles of the Central Highlands of Vietnam and if there was any reason he made it home alive, believing that God had delivered him out of that hell was as good as any other. It wasn't that he abandoned his German Lutheran upbringing. He just saw too much and did too much during the war to leave the faith of his youth unscathed.

A man could cling to his religion, but the bush was tough on one's untested beliefs. The Ten Commandments he grew up with were attacked by the dispassionate reality of killing and dying. After the fight, the violence had a way of slowly corroding whatever survived first contact. Faith, fate, life, and death were rearranged by the war's uncaring calculus, leaving one to make sense of the broken shards. That crucifix helped him reassemble the pieces. And now it was gone.

Don's unit, the 3/12th, was always on the move. But the longer they occupied a position, the more effort they put into fortifying themselves

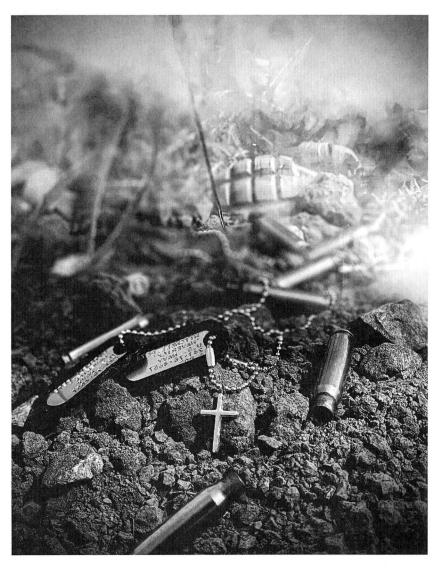

Author's photograph.

against what was coming. As a mortar man, that meant bigger and deeper mortar pits. Nothing replaced good cover. For the exhausted troops, the costly balance of toil and survival in combat was a constant struggle.

That day, they arrived at their new position and were ordered to dig in on the top of a ridge overlooking the dense jungle below. Don and his mortar section were digging their new pit next to a towering tree. They were hacking at its broad trunk with machetes, the only inadequate tool available for such a job. It was draining work. Their waiting 81mm ammo supply sat stacked on the earthen floor of the shallow pit while they took turns with the dulled blades, determined to clear their fire lane of the tree's obstructing canopy.

In the distance, the beating of helicopter blades echoed off the mountain walls. Like a dinner bell, the Huey's sound signature lured men's attention from everywhere. It might be food, water, ammo, or other desperately needed supplies, but it wouldn't have been coming to this God-forsaken mountain without something important.

It was the red mail bags kicked out the door that drew the biggest crowds. Men were desperate for anything from "the world." A letter, or better yet, a care package, may bring the only joy a man could muster so far from home.

Don and his mortar team perked at the sound of the inbound chopper. They had enough time in the bush to decipher the message of the blade pitch, the increasing volume, and the heading. In unison, and without a word, they stopped hacking at the base of the tree next to their unfinished mortar pit and silently made their way towards the top of the mountain. The combat engineers who created the fresh LZ on its crest were clearing the last of the felled trees.

As the chopper approached, weary olive-clad men emerged out of the jungle. They were hopeful, but learned not to confuse that with certainty. Experience taught them to stay stoic—better to stay indifferent than feel the pain of crushed expectations.

Besides, occasionally, those red bags held a "Dear John" letter. It was hard watching a man's desperate need for comfort from home crumble as his girl explained her reasons she wouldn't be waiting for his return.

That day, there were no red bags. There were only the familiar OD green wooden crates. The yellow stenciling stolidly noted the type of encased ammunition that kept it all going: more shooting, more killing, more dying.

But before the Huey crew and some grunts unloaded the crates, a solitary man stepped out of the door holding down the lip of his helmet against the red whirlwind of dusty rotor wash. He caught everyone's attention because he didn't look like the rest of them.

The man carried no weapon, wore no web gear, and substituted a small satchel bag for a rucksack. And he didn't carry himself like the others; his stride conveyed an air of assurance that hadn't been humbled by the jungle. His uniform remained the deep OD green that the men of the 3/12th were once issued. Months in the penetrating sun, mud, and corrosive elements transformed their battlefield utilities into varying shades of bleached earth tones and tattered filth.

The onlookers were jungle fighters who noticed the slightest thing out of place. The stranger's glaring contrast piqued their curiosity. What was this untested, defenseless man doing out in the middle of hell? The question needed an answer.

Don peered at the odd newcomer as he carried the bag in one hand while holding his steel pot down with the other. He shimmied beyond the radius of the helicopter's dust storm, before standing straight and meeting the company commander's aides. Don watched as they shook hands in a hurried introduction before pointing the unarmed man to a part of the freshly created LZ. A large, sheared stump bore the scars of the det cord used to take down the tree it once belonged to.

The man set the bag down on the stump and removed his helmet. He unzipped it, removed the embroidered stole and reverently placed it upon his shoulders. From the bag, he carefully removed his bible and rosary which he brought to his lips before laying them by the gold cross which he had erected on his makeshift table.

Motionless, Don and his mortar crew watched the chaplain prepare to bring the word of God to this soulless place.

After methodical preparation, the leader of this impromptu service gently turned his arms up in praise as he looked to the heavens. Don glanced at his best friend, Garitt, fellow mortar man and devout Catholic, and smiled. The gathering crowd of soldiers sensed the wordless call to prayer and filtered through the brush towards the invisible church.

If there was a divine presence in Vietnam, there was no sign of it. Don humped the bush too long. He'd seen too much death. God or no God, he never knew if he would live through the day. When he saw tomorrow, he'd dread dusk and repeated the process with each rising sun. But he also knew another truism of war; there are no atheists in foxholes.

Don and his team reverently took a knee as the chaplain offered the invocation of the collect to start his service. The liturgy wove in God's grace and their absolution from their necessary deeds of war.

The service didn't last long. In the boonies, God would have to understand that bunching up for that long was a mistake no matter what the reason. Don had lost count of how often the new guys had to be reminded to spread the hell out. It was always followed by the ominous reminder—one round would get you all.

After a closing prayer, the chaplain reached into his bag and passed out small golden crucifixes to his hastily assembled congregation. Don removed the chain holding his dog tags and his P38 can opener, and threaded the tag end through the cross's metal loop.

When he put that crucifix around his neck, he couldn't know that he would survive the war, and would wear this cross for the next fifty years. He also had no idea how quickly he would need its protective power.

The congregated warriors lingered in the comfort of the service and the man who had risked his life to come out to the war to offer it to them. They milled about while some of the troops sought a brief, private moment with this man of God. There was no time to discuss their suffering. They would have struggled to put it into words even if there was. They settled for the fleeting aura of sanctuary offered by this man of the cloth.

For a few quiet moments, Don peered down at the cross. His mind sought refuge in the past of what seemed like another lifetime.

He revisited his hometown church and especially the warm candlelit glow of the Christmas service. He felt the innocent embrace of his childhood when the only wars he knew of were in movies. The soldiers, after being killed on screen, got up, dusted off, and were granted another day. Don reveled in that time when he felt so safe and protected, and didn't know there was any other way to live.

The chaplain's congregants were not the only soldiers who heard the inbound chopper. They, too, had been in the bush long enough to translate the Huey's heading and calculate the location of its destination.

Don's childhood daydream back home was suddenly shattered by the distant thump of mortars leaving their tubes. His team suddenly jolted into the alarming present. The ominous whistling followed a few moments later. Men chaotically scurried in every direction to take cover.

"Incoming!! Move! MOVE IT!!"

The random death of mortars was terrifying as there was no logical defense; one could only hide in a hole or behind something and pray one did not land near you. If caught in the open, a man could only get as low to the ground as possible to avoid the deadly cone of searing shrapnel that would slice through anything above knee height. The deafening blast and bone-jarring concussion made a man curse the buttons on his jungle shirt for not allowing him to get closer to the ground.

The enemy developed an uncanny knack for knowing where assets would be positioned inside the American infantry perimeter. The first volley struck to the east of the LZ. The chain of explosions walked across the ridge line where Don and his crew dug their mortar pit.

A massive secondary explosion shook the earth. A huge fireball boiled into the air as shrapnel peppered the surrounding jungle. Don watched the tree they were chopping down earlier became engulfed in flame and billowing black smoke. Its burning trunk lurched to one side and gradually accelerated until it crashed into the forest.

The attack didn't last long. When the enemy faced a superior force, it rarely did. They would strike like lightning before dissolving back into the dense surrounding highlands.

Don's instincts told him this was such a time. It ended as quickly as it began. His guys policed up their gear and cautiously approached the ridgeline. They headed for the felled tree that only twenty minutes earlier was their nemesis. The stump and surrounding brush were still burning, the smoke congealing into a pulsating dark column that dirtied the low cumulus cloud cover. Glowing embers wafted through the air like ominous fireflies. It was then they discovered that their freshly dug pit full of tubes of prepared and armed 81mm rounds had taken a direct hit.

Don stared at the smoldering crater in the red earth he and his team had occupied only a short time ago. His eyes tracked the circular zone of destruction left by the blast radius. The surrounding trees were splintered, their foliage shredded. His lips trembled as he realized how very close they all had come.

Then it hit him.

Don reached for his dog tag chain and pulled it out of his sour olive drab tee shirt. Its pristine finish shone against his soiled hand. Had he not gone to the chaplain's service, he and his men would still have been working on taking down that tree. He chalked up the other brushes with death to luck. But this time it was unmistakable; an ordained messenger hand delivered it to him.

He stared at the crucifix and pressed it tightly in his palm as he bowed his head in a swirl of gratitude and the stark recognition of how close he had come to his young end once again. It was, to him, also an omen; he was forgiven for whatever he had done in the bush to make it home alive. Those painful secrets were now between him and God.

In Vietnam, if a man didn't have something to believe in, he'd have to find or create it. However, this message was delivered to him as surely as a letter from one of those red bags on the chopper.

It worked. His heavenly Father now had his attention.

Don cherished his cross. It was now the epicenter of not only his faith, but the guarantor of his soldier's luck. Without something to hold on to, a man was subject to the overwhelming forces of darkness arrayed against him. No matter one's religious beliefs, most in the field believed that when your luck ran out … well, it was just your time.

Because of this, Don understood his First Sergeant's anguish the day he lost his own heirloom crucifix in the jungle.

It was just like any other patrol in Vietnam. The 3/12th was walking the endless trails snaking through the mountainous jungle in search of the enemy. However, this time, they were in company strength and Don was traveling with the last of four platoons in the long column on another timeless march.

The corpulent First Sergeant had no business in the bush. He was a base camp cook who had never fired a shot in anger, but he was short and didn't want to leave Vietnam without his CIB—proof that he had been in the shit. But he was too old and overweight to be humping with a line company. And everybody knew it.

He couldn't keep up with others on his best day. By the time he suddenly realized the familiar sensation of his gold chain around his neck was gone, he had already fallen back near the tail end of the serpentine column. Don saw his panicked sweat-covered face as the Sergeant rifled through his flak vest and web gear.

"It's gone! I have to go back.... I have to find it!"

Don reached for the reassuring dog tag chain around his neck. He felt the stinging terror in the Sergeant's voice. It was the fright of a man who discovered that his shield was gone, exposing him to the darkness of the jungle's omnipresent evil. The Sergeant's labored breathing from hours on the move accelerated as he turned and started back down the trail they just created through the dense underbrush.

Don called after him in a loud whisper.

"Sarge! We are already falling behind ... you gotta let it go. We have to keep up with the others!"

But it was too late—he couldn't let it go. Don was already losing sight of the Sergeant barreling through the foliage as its branches briefly parted only to swallow him as he passed. Don followed him before reaching the last few bewildered troops pulling rear guard.

In pursuit, he stopped to grab the shoulder straps of the very last man to get his attention.

"Where is he?!?" he blurted out between his gasping breaths. "The First Sergeant who passed you.... Where?!?"

The rear guard looked incredulously at the fools heading the wrong way. He had been in country too long to care anymore beyond cracking a smirk. He pointed towards the dense jungle wall behind him.

Don followed the fading trail pausing every twenty meters to listen. He glanced back in the direction of the company, whose protection drifted further away. Don fought the smothering fear of being lost in this feral wilderness, but it only grew with every step.

The narrow trail he was struggling to follow was closing up as if the land were devouring them alive. Soon, he no longer heard the hurried steps of the panic-fueled Sergeant. Don stopped again and strained to hear. There was nothing but the indifferent native chorus of the jungle.

He was torn, but his instincts made the final call. He had spent too much time trying to survive to make any other decision. Don resolutely turned and then double timed it back up the trail.

Within minutes, reassuring glimpses of the rear element appeared accompanied by unmistakable sounds of exhausted grunts humping the bush.

Don continued up the trail until he found the Lieutenant to report the missing man. The officer briefly considered the situation, but even before he gave his orders, Don knew the cold facts—the mission came before the man. The Lieutenant assured that when they reached their destination, he would report the missing man to the Captain.

Then, they moved on.

But Don couldn't move on. He felt his crucifix resting just above his heart. The haunting image of the panicked Sergeant desperately looking for his in the jungle swirled through his mind. He sensed the gnawing grip of emotions he didn't want to feel.

When they set up camp at dusk, he impatiently sought out the Captain's RTO and pressed him for information.

"They sent the Rangers after him. If he's out there, they'll find him," the RTO assured.

The Rangers were good, but Don knew the terrain too well. The steep grade of the mountains and the unpredictable weather alone could kill even a well-conditioned man. The inhospitable jungle was filled with a gauntlet of predators of every genus. Only weeks ago, they had lost a man in 2nd platoon to a tiger attack. Don listened in helpless horror as the screams fell silent and grisly sounds of the kill wafted through the jungle. Out in the bush, you could count yourself lucky if the land alone spared you.

Don kept asking, but never learned if the Rangers found his First Sergeant. It was just one more man who appeared briefly during his tour whose unknown fate disappeared into the war's infinite apathy.

Don visited the Vietnam Veterans Memorial Wall before but couldn't bring himself to look for the First Sergeant's name. While he never heard word if the Rangers found him, he couldn't bear the thought that he was the last man to see him alive.

But it wasn't just whether he was dead or alive.

It was that choice. That awful choice.

Don knew how his fellow troops addressed such stark dilemmas in the field, but it didn't help him feel better about it. Everyone out there thought it, even if only a few actually said it—better him than me.

After coming home, that calloused realism had no place in the civilized world. The bitter truth of that fact only made him feel worse. No one understood the burden he now carried. For that reason, Sarge's fate stayed buried in shallow graves for decades along with too many other things he didn't want to remember.

After the war, like so many other cordoned memories, Don found life mock his efforts to steer clear of their painful reminders. They were everywhere. And in an instant, he suddenly found himself back in the jungle.

There was that time his daughter eyed something special at the mall. When she brought him to the jewelry department in a pitch for its purchase, he felt the stir of old ghosts. He looked into the brightly lit case and saw the golden crucifix on its 14-karat chain before the case began to dim, and then went black.

"Dad? Are you OK?"

Her voice echoed as if in a tunnel. When the blur focused again, Don saw her face, wearing fearful curiosity as only a daughter could. He felt a bead of sweat drip from his forehead before it was intercepted by his thick gray brow. The walls began closing in before he grabbed her hand and headed for the exit.

He couldn't explain it to her just yet. Don promised himself that he would talk to her about the war when she turned sixteen, but that milestone came and went. He still struggled with what to say and how to say it. So he didn't.

The hard truth was that he didn't know how to explain it to himself. He brought it into his therapy session and we unpacked his dissociative episode at the mall. Before that session, he had never talked about the First Sergeant and the decision he had to make in the jungle that day. He wrestled through that painful memory and placed it along side of the many others he was working through. It was a slow, uneven process, but Don was beginning to heal.

~

Don searched everywhere, but it was nowhere to be found. It was just another day of running errands. As he walked through the parking lot, a jolt of awareness stopped him in his tracks. Though his mind was focused on his next stop, part of him detected the absence of the sensation around his neck that had been a part of his life for fifty-one years. It was his protector during the war and physical reminder of his connection to the divine.

And now it was gone.

That night, his ghosts couldn't ignore the rhyme and came to visit once again. Don tossed and involuntarily jerked in his sleep as he saw himself lost in the bush chasing Sarge as the jungle wrapped itself around him like a serpent's coils. He awoke in the smothering darkness with a start, sitting straight up in bed. His bedclothes were soaked with sweat, his body thumping in alarm by the vivid replaying of that day in the jungle.

Still disoriented, he stumbled to the bathroom and, in the faint glow of the nightlight, splashed some cold water on his face. With still trembling fingers, he fumbled for his pill bottle before emptying a capsule into his clammy hand. He chased it with some water and took a deep breath as he braced himself on the edge of the vanity. The nightmare, though further away, continued to loop. He soon felt the medicine creep into his system, bringing its welcomed calm.

For years, after his nightmares, Don went straight to the liquor cabinet and poured himself a few fingers before trying to retire again. He was trying to change that approach, went to the couch, put the TV on softly, and patiently waited. He eventually felt his body relax and his eyelids drop. He changed his shirt, and, with some trepidation, climbed back into bed.

His demons weren't done yet. Eyes undulated beneath his lids trying to escape going back. Suddenly, he found himself in the dim triple canopy jungle on a mountain trail. Alone.

Though he was in jungle fatigues, he looked down at his thick forearms covered in gray hair and his protruding belly. He recognized his seventy-one-year-old body and became uncannily aware that he was, at once, himself but on the same trail and in the same predicament as the old First Sergeant was so many years ago. The panic jolted through him as he struggled to catch his breath. Only now it was now his cross that was lost. In front of him, the carnivorous jaws of the jungle opened with a sinister hiss.

~

The morning after his nightmare, Don called to process the chilling brush with his past triggered by the loss of his crucifix.

He shared this story and we cleaved towards the work he needed to do, looking for the message he now needed to receive. But first, there was an old question that first needed answering before we could figure out which path he needed to take.

"Do you want to know?"

"I think it's time. Yes…. I need to know."

It didn't take but a few minutes on the virtual Vietnam Veterans Memorial Wall website to answer the fifty-one-year-old question.

"He's not there, Don. Your First Sergeant is not on the Wall."

The relief through the phone line was palpable.

"OK…so unless he officially went MIA, that means he made it."

We sat with that new, hopeful story. Though I could not see his face, I could feel the gears turning in his mind. Then, the insight effortlessly poured out of him.

"So maybe, I just need to let it go. Maybe losing my cross happened for that reason. If God wants me to find it, I will. I need to trust that. He brought me the crucifix to save me that day on that mountain with the chaplain, and maybe it's gone now for the same reason. And I know I did what I could to find the First Sergeant without sacrificing my own life. I think I just need to let the guilt go with it and turn it over to Him."

That day, Don let both of his crosses go. We sat in silent reverence as that epiphany sunk in for us both.

A month later, Don found his crucifix.

28

Well of Forgiveness

He sat before me trying to figure out how to answer a simple, but not so simple question.

"Hmmm. How am I?"

Jack didn't rush his answer and his eyes suggested moments of honest soul searching. He smiled.

"I am OK. I'm really OK. I would say I am content and comfortable."

I had no doubt that he meant what he said. He'd done a tremendous amount of emotional work to get here. I didn't say it with words, but my expression did. It was filled with pride for his hard-fought peace. His smile broadened a little more and though he did not hear me say it, I didn't have to.

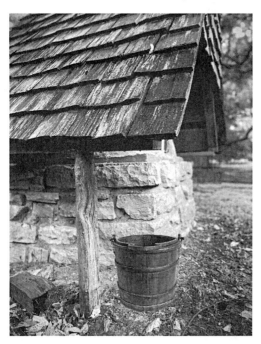

Author's photograph.

He got it.

Jack sat silently, waiting for the right words to express themselves.

"I've been thinking a lot about who I am now and reflecting on the mistakes I made earlier in my life before, during, and since Vietnam."

He struggled like all young boys to find the man inside of themselves they hoped to become. He left home earlier than many. But in some ways, Jack was

216

lucky. Angels appeared at the right times to help guide him through the tough spots that no one else bothered to show up for. Sometimes, that fleeting luck became another hard lesson. When he had nowhere else to go, an old sheriff and justice of the peace took him in as a guest on his ranch. Soon, he too, had to draw the line and ask Jack to leave.

Jack savored the kindness of these unexpected supporters and felt the sting of their departures. He longed for their kindness, love, and guidance to help salve the deepest wound from his childhood—that he was not good enough, and unworthy of redemption and forgiveness for his misdeeds.

In his therapy, we worked on those early lies and he began to heal. He came to appreciate the truth of who he was then and now, but those early injuries still hurt when he touched them. We pivoted to the deep work he was doing in his recent return to one of my PTSD groups.

In those sessions, when Jack spoke, his soul poured into the room. The group sat, transfixed in silence, admiring the raw vulnerability, passion, and honesty on display. For men vigilant for the same lies they heard too many times before, they didn't need to be sold; when Jack spoke, they felt the unmistakable presence of truth.

And they needed it now more than ever.

The group was working on one of the last, but most important, inner destinations combat veterans care to visit—their guilt and shame. Because of the agony, we would often get to this topic by accident, because it was too closely guarded to get there on purpose. Even then, it took courage to stay. Like in combat, the safety of the group helped them venture into their fear—together.

We could hear the anguish in his voice. What they couldn't, or didn't want to see in themselves, Jack showed them in reflection. They contemplated if there was a way—any way, out of the corrosiveness of a guilty conscious.

I surveyed the room during such an uncomfortable silence. Men twisted in their chairs, legs bouncing. We were getting close.

We came too far to get here and I wasn't about to let them leave empty-handed. For some, it was the first time. For others, a return to shallow graves. We searched for a way through. Along the way, they revisited all of the familiar dead ends … raging, drinking, fighting, numbing, hiding, running….

They spent decades pushing against their own walls in search of escape, hoping they would collapse through sheer force of will. But they were older, weary, and too wise for that now. They needed another answer, and eventually found one.

It was the same path that many before them discovered when nothing else worked—forgiveness. Jack saw it clearly now, but only because of his hellish journey required to retrieve it. His two combat tours in Vietnam with the 173rd Airborne were a horrendous price to pay for that sacred knowledge. He felt it his duty to pass it on.

As we sat in my office continuing our session, Jack looked up as if to retrieve something invisible hovering above us. He then returned to my eyes.

"I have a story about forgiveness that could possibly help the group."

He began speaking and we both let go of the present, tumbling into the jungle-booted footprints of his past.

Jack's gut twisted in response to the descending Huey. Though the Lieutenant advised the enemy wasn't in the area, the reaction came anyway. He briefed the squad over the whirl of the accelerating turbine. The LZ was cold, but friendlies were on the ground questioning prisoners.

The thatched roofs of the village of Phu Hiep-2 appeared beneath the low cloud cover. The bucolic image disappeared in the tornadic rotor wash pressing into the red earth. Airborne infantry jumped from the skids holding the brims of their faded boonie hats as they scurried beyond the dusty funnel. They fanned out to set up a security perimeter as the fading rhythm of the ascending chopper's blades gave way to the sound of wailing.

Wiping the dusty grim from his eyes, he tried to focus on the fuzzy forms in the town square. Jack couldn't believe what he saw.

His voice shook and his tear-filled eyes widened drawing me into his horror. I braced myself for what I sensed was coming. His head dropped and his hands shook as he assembled the scene.

The screams zeroed Jack's attention to a tight cluster of tiger-striped South Vietnamese troops by the village well. He recognized their insignias as Special Police, and knew of their reputation. Standing off to the right were two Americans without unit patches.

Jack felt his gut tighten. He figured they were CIA supervising the interrogations. He knew their reputation, too. Then he heard it.

Sounds of medieval struggle—gurgling … choking … gasping.

On the ground, beyond the fence of tiger-striped legs, sat two wailing forms clinging to one another as they watched the pair of thrashing bare feet visible from behind the stone wall.

Jack panned the faces of his squad, but saw nothing but blank stares of men who had already seen too much. In horror, he stood alone.

He turned back to scowls of men towering over their captives—shouting, laughing. Another furiously turned the squeaking metal handle until it raised another splashing bucket of well water, before handing it to the pair kneeling over the prisoner. One pulled the muslin rag pulled tightly across her gagging mouth as the other poured a steady stream into it. The sickening gurgle began again as helpless legs fought to find air.

The high-pitched wail began again.

"Mẹ! ... Mẹ!!"

Jack translated but I didn't need to understand Vietnamese to know what he witnessed that day at Phu Hiep-2. Men whom Jack referred to as "friendlies" were waterboarding a young mother in front of her two children.

Jack tried to appeal to the young paratrooper closest to him, but found he was alone. Morality had long ago given way to what was necessary. If one could do that long enough out in the bush, there was a better chance he may go home.

"It's none of our business. If you can't look, go on the other side of that tree."

The details were so gut wrenching and so monolithic, I became enveloped in the story's dark evocative power. As he narrated, we both sat in suspension somewhere between those two worlds. I could no longer hear the ticking second hand of the wall clock over his right shoulder, and anchors of time and space fell away.

There was only his story—he shared it, and I listened; I did so with the full depth of my being. We were bound by the tether of trust between us, and that alone created the only available assurance needed to continue our descent into this hellish vortex.

He continued....

"Our squad was then ordered out. As we walked down the trail out of the Ville, we heard three shots. By the time we made it back, there was no one to be found. After some searching, we found their three bodies. They dumped them down the village well."

As he described the macabre discovery, the sadness and regret poured out of him. The smallest of their squad, Rat, shimmied down the well's stone walls to retrieve the bodies. They went to a berm on the edge of the village and buried the slain mother and her two children. Then, like the soldiers they were trained to be, they saddled up and moved on to their next objective.

But Jack never moved on.

He endured many horrors of war during his tour as an infantryman until he was wounded, and later returned for a second tour as a combat photographer. But a piece of him would forever remain buried with those bodies in that village.

And that was precisely why he had to go back.

"That's what my worst nightmares were about—I would have many variations … in the dreams, I would try to do something different. I would take action that I didn't take that day. In one, I would shoot the interrogators. In another, I would shoot the three prisoners to put them out of the misery of their torture. But no matter what I did, the nightmares persisted and so did my guilt."

In the years following, Jack tried to find a way to come to terms with the way the war lived in him, but nothing seemed to work. A final option remained. He needed to go back. He needed to go back to Vietnam. That's where the ghosts were….

Only Jack didn't just go back. He moved his entire family to Hanoi where he taught English. He lived among and befriended his former enemy, and hoped that this experience of connection and penance would free his tortured conscious. And it did … for a while.

He tried to answer the unrelenting hurt by looking somewhere else— anywhere else. He traveled the entire country trying to find the peace that eluded him. Mostly, he found acceptance and friendship. Slowly, with each place he visited, his experiences with the Vietnamese fortified his nascent courage. He would need it.

While each of those travels were important, he was avoiding the one that was critical. Jack knew that the place he needed to go was the very place he feared going most of all.

The gravitational pull of Phu Hiep-2 beckoned him. Jack eventually surrendered to it, making the 603-mile journey to Phú Yên province in South Vietnam. He felt the coming confrontation with his demons intensify as he made his way down QL28, the dusty road leading him into the scene of his nightmares.

Upon arriving in the small village, he anxiously surveyed the grounds. He could scarcely believe how little it had changed since the war and its sameness blurred the moment with overwhelming images. He began to shake and cry.

An old man observed the emotional round-eyed stranger, clearly out of place, and calmly approached him. Customary pleasantries gave way to the immediate intimacy formed by Jack's raw despair. He couldn't look the elder villager in the face; the man's weathered features and gray hair signaled he was old enough to have been there when the sky soldiers set up their perimeter on the edge of the village that day. That mere possibility amplified his guilt and his fear to unimaginable heights.

Overwhelmed into silence, tears streamed down Jack's cheeks. The old man's assuring grace only intensified his weeping, but also helped him open his mouth enough to pull the central question through his quivering lips.

"Can you forgive me?" he begged.

"For what?" the old man inquired.

"I can't tell you!" Jack wailed. "Can you *just* forgive me?"

The elder reached out to him and, with an ethereal touch, invited him into his nearby home. There he sat Jack down as his honored guest, poured them both a cup of steaming green tea and, with tenderness and reassurance, peered deep into Jack's eyes.

"...được rồi ...It's okay," the man softly invited. "Tell me your story."

Jack summoned the strength to tell a safer version of his most guarded secret. His shame filled the room after he narrated the last time he was in this village. Through tear-filled eyes, he again begged for forgiveness.

"Why do you ask for my forgiveness?" the old man asked with incredulity. "Why? Forgive you for what?"

The old man's utter lack of judgment breached his last line of resistance. How many times had he thought it over years? How many times had it shown itself on the marquis of his guilty conscious? Yet never had these words passed his lips. He felt the truth rising to liberate itself. Finally, came its merciful death.

"Because.... Because I did nothing! I watched it happen and I did *nothing!*"

Its collapse in the face of the old man's acceptance created the courage for him to tell the whole story. He shared the agonizing truths of that day he flew into Phu Hiep-2. He told him of the horror he saw. He told him of the torture and killings. He admitted how that day took his American morals and humanity, and smashed them upon the earth on which they sat.

Jack was dizzied by the whirlwind of relief and shame. He sat in bafflement, unable to understand the villager's response to his confession; it simply didn't fit with what Jack was certain would be the same disgust and condemnation with which he had tortured himself for so many years. His nakedness stared at the floor, waiting.

But it never came. Jack had to look once more to make sure he wasn't desperately imposing his wish for redemption on the moment. Cautiously, he raised his eyes.

In front of him sat the old man, his face beaming with light, gratitude and love.

"You came to our village seeking forgiveness for doing *nothing*? You have done *everything!*" the old man said with joy.

Jack's brows wrinkled in disbelief, trying to make sense out the old man's radiance.

"I don't... I don't understand...."

The old man beamed, and explained the *real* reason he came back to visit Phu Hiep-2. The man, who was the elder chieftain of his war-torn village then told his story:

His people settled and lived in this valley in Phú Yên province for the last 1,500 years. Their country had seen many invaders and centuries of war. The day the sky soldiers came to this place so many years ago, the entire village had been cleared of all inhabitants; some were killed, some arrested, some relocated, and some were never heard from again. After the war, many survivors returned home to resume their lives, but the land and its people were wounded.

The village, he explained, remained unhealed all of these years. Particularly painful were those who suddenly disappeared without a trace and could not be laid to rest with their ancestors as their traditions required. The elder then looked at Jack who was desperately trying to make sense out of their surreal encounter. A merciful clarity came next.

"During that time, my daughter and my two grandchildren disappeared and were never found. Don't you see? You came to our village today to bring them back to us!"

Jack was not sure how to feel. He sat, stunned by the inconceivable serendipity of this revelation. He was dizzied by what he just heard, for it was opposite of everything he believed and felt down to the core of his being for so long.

This man, whose daughter and grandchildren were murdered and thrown down a well by men who had worn the same uniform as he, was overjoyed by this momentous reunification. This man lived so long with the gaping loss of not knowing, now knew; his loved ones and their souls were finally coming home.

Jack showed the old man the berm of laterite earth and burial site where he and his squad tried to amend the great wrong they witnessed. Word of this mystery's end spread throughout the village and then, the entire valley.

Hundreds of Viet people, dressed in white, emerged and descended on the village of Phu Hiep-2. They celebrated the return of their lost loved ones, and the miracle of the arrival of the sky soldier who came seeking forgiveness, but completed a critical chapter in the village's collective pain and fractured ancestral history. This former enemy brought healing to the people and the land. Then, the remains of the missing were lovingly tended to and laid to final rest.

Jack left the village of Phu Hiep-2 a different man. He touched the true meaning of forgiveness; it had been wrapped around him like a loving blanket. The account was settled. He never had the nightmare of what he witnessed that day in the village again.

Jack sat looking at me and I at him. Though he had told some isolated pieces of that story before, I never heard the entire account. I sat stunned by the horrific pain, it's perfect synchronicity, and its unimaginable redemption.

It was a near biblical account of forgiveness … and it was not over. Jack continued….

"When I got back to Hanoi in late 1994, I learned they were demolishing the 'Maison Centrale' prison." This was yet another place Jack felt the irresistible gravity of the painful past.

Built in the 1880s by the French colonial government to detain Vietnamese political prisoners, the name in French translated to "Central House." In Vietnamese, it is called "Hỏa Lò." It is better known to Americans as the "Hanoi Hilton" and was the infamous primary facility in which American POWs were tortured and imprisoned during the war.

When Jack arrived at Hỏa Lò, behind the tall exterior walls topped with cemented broken glass, arose the drone of heavy equipment and the sound of crumpling bricks. The interior structures were already falling to the wrecking ball, as if to collapse the only standing testament of Vietnamese perfidy during the war.* The dust of the past rose in escape over the walls and filtered into the indifference of the bordering street.

Due to the horrors that lived behind these walls, it was simultaneously a testament to the courage and fortitude of many American servicemen who suffered inside of them and survived years of harsh captivity. Jack wanted to be there to witness its destruction.

As he tried to find a way to access this hallowed place of American bravery, he encountered a Vietnamese man about his age in front of the prison. Jack inquired as to how he might get in for a closer look.

"Come back here at five o'clock tonight," The man said. "By then, they will be done for the day."

The man appeared sincere and Jack did exactly as advised.

At five that evening, he returned to silence on the other side of the wall and knocked on the heavy door of the arched main entrance. A moment later, the man who instructed him earlier stood outlined in the doorway. Jack reflexively stepped back before the fear hit him.

The man was wearing military greens and a red star-adorned pith helmet—the uniform of his former enemy. The man offered an assuring hand to meet Jack's recoil and beckoned him inside the prison gate.

With a confusing echo to Phu Hiep-2, Jack wasn't sure how to feel in that moment. His instincts screamed at him as he stood in front of a man resembling his enemy in the physical epicenter of their hatred for Jack and his brothers in arms. Yet his instant read detected no threat.

Oddly, he sensed this he needed to follow this man. As the man smiled, turned and waved him forward, Jack yielded to his gut and cautiously trailed him through some halls and into the prison's crumbling courtyard.

The deconstruction was well underway and the pea green stucco of

C-block, which once imprisoned Senator John McCain as well as other senior U.S. airmen, lay in partial ruin. The quiet testimony of narrow cells spoke through the scattered mounds of brick. Jack stared at their outlines of his comrades' agony on the other side of the now-half demolished walls. Tears blurred his vision as he turned inward to fight against the emotional tsunami engulfing his body.

He startled as he felt light touch on his shoulder. It shocked him into the present as if he had been struck by a bolt of lightning.

Behind him stood the uniformed man reaching out to him. In his hand was a nine-pound sledgehammer, offering to the man he once considered an invader.

"...được rồi … it's okay … take it."

He pointed with permission towards the remaining brick wall of C-block.

Jack slowly reached for the hammer and once in his hands, the anger waiting for such a moment welded his clenched hands to its worn wooden handle. He swung the hammer and a section of the wall shattered under the full force of his rage. As he did so, he imagined liberating the spirits of all who had withered behind it. He continued to swing the sledge over and over as if their collective anguish powered his every blow.

Jack dropped it at his feet, and bent over, heaving for air. Having exhausted every ounce of strength he could muster, he paused to catch his breath and prepared for another assault on the mangled wall. In his blind fury, he had momentarily lost awareness of his guide.

Behind him, the uniformed man stood silently, but impatiently. His face had shifted to an expression that Jack had trouble placing. He appeared to be wrestling with his own feelings, but Jack couldn't be sure. He instinctively extended the hammer to the man wondering if he, too, had something he desperately needed to release.

The man held up his hands in refusal as if to fight the truth he feared the hammer may find. Besides, the prison was surrounded by tall apartment buildings and he knew the consequences of any unchecked emotional display was reportable as an "unpatriotic act" to his communist government. However, his protestations were but a thin levy against the flood of feelings welling up from deep within him.

Jack studied the man's face and saw the moment he surrendered to the truth he could no longer keep buried. His head sunk in shame. The tears streamed down his face and he paused one last moment before he slowly raised his head and looked deep into Jack's eyes.

"Will you forgive me?" he pleaded. "Please … forgive me…!"

Jack looked at him with disbelief. "Forgive *you*? Forgive you for *what*?"

The man contemplated the great risk of telling his secret to this American stranger—his former enemy. He recognized that the universe was providing this single chance. A chance to reconcile. Perhaps the only one he would ever have to square his karmic account. When he realized there would never be another moment like this, his courage appeared. His rising, trembling arm led the way to the truth.

"Do you see that door over there?"

Jack looked behind him. It was the same door the man led him through into the courtyard not an hour ago. He nodded in assent.

"During the war, that door was my post. It was my job to check visitors' paperwork before allowing them entry into Hỏa Lò."

As the man narrated his brief story, the tears continued to stream down his face. That, however, was not his big secret. Jack knew that fear. The tension rose as the man worked his way towards the real story behind his curious request for absolution. The pauses stretched as he got closer.

Jack still didn't understand, but took a deep breath. He noticed the emerging, translucent image of the village chieftain of Phu Hiep-2, his eyes radiating grace. Jack's furrowed brow melted into a serene gaze. A gentle swell of calm washed over him. Sensing safety, the man let go, and plunged into his darkness.

"While I was at that door, I heard them! I heard everything...." The man confessed as he wept. "I heard them torturing the Americans ... and I did nothing! I did *nothing....* Please ... forgive me!" He dropped his head as decades of pain poured from him.

On this day, Jack and the man, mere strangers on opposing sides of history, joined in their wounding; their pain over the war, for what they did during it and, very importantly, what they *didn't* do. And they healed.

Jack never forgot this day. Or this man he did not know. During that surreal encounter, the man selected one of the bricks from the wall of C-block, wrote his name on the bottom of the brick, and then set it down on the ground to embrace the American who had accompanied him to the grave of his secret, and helped liberate him. The embrace lasted—it had too. Both sensed this would be the first, and only time they would meet. It was.

When Jack turned to retrieve the personalized memento, a white pigeon was perched on the signed brick and when it launched to flight, it left behind a single ivory feather.

Jack sat across from me, smiling as he finished his story with an omen of peace, reconciliation, and forgiveness. His tears from this profoundly moving descent into his darkest corners of his being had not yet started to dry.

"I still have that brick and feather," Jack stated with a tear-framed smile.

I sat in awe of this stunning story. It was the most incredible tale of forgiveness and healing I had ever heard. After Jack left session that day, I reflected on the profundity of not only the gut wrenching but beautiful story, but the equally wrenching and beautiful journey I had just taken with this man I have grown to care for deeply.

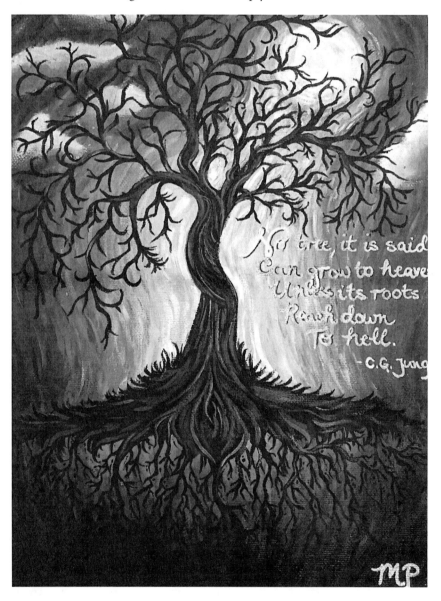

Student's gift of Tree of Life (author's collection).

It was then it hit me.

In my office, behind my chair, hangs a hand-painted art piece. It was a gift from a former student with whom I had worked closely. She had a great appreciation for the nature of my work and my unwavering dedication to our combat veterans in trauma recovery. The subject of the painting was chosen carefully with this in mind.

It depicts the tree of life—its branches touch a clouded but sun-kissed sky while the roots reach into the fire of the underworld. The painted caption is a quote of Dr. Carl Jung, a pioneer psychoanalyst.

It reads, "No tree, it is said, can grow to heaven unless its roots reach down to hell."

I thought I appreciated the meaning of that painting; however, I would not fully feel what that meant as I did the day I heard this story. Then, the title of this yet-unwritten story came as a crystal-clear awareness rather than a thought....

*In 2016 when I personally visited Hỏa Lò prison and met Colonel Duyệt, the commandant of the prison during the war, he flatly denied any torture of American POWs occurred at all on his watch.

29

War Smiles

His wide smile echoed the grinning Vietnamese boy draped over his tanned, shirtless torso. Though unarmed and donning a pair of sandals, his sun-bleached jungle utility trousers and matching soft cover on his head reminded him that the smiles hid a darker truth—these were not happy times.

Fifty-two years later, the oxidizing photo was the only remaining evidence that Michael had anything to smile about during that war.

Though I was his therapist, I would have never seen this image had it not been for my trip to Vietnam in the fall of 2016. Upon learning I was accompanying a group of Vietnam veterans back to the once–war torn

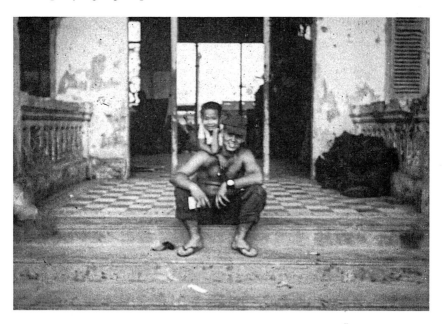

Soldier of 15th Engineers with local boy, Bến Tre, RVN (veteran photograph).

country for a healing and reconciliation journey with the organization Soldier's Heart, Michael asked about our itinerary. I flipped through the travel packet and ticked off the list of destinations.

His jaw dropped and eyes widened before I got halfway through.

"Wait ... you're going to Bến Tre?" he half-asked, half-stated. Michael's inflection spoke volumes of his connection with that place.

I looked back at the name that meant nothing to me, and everything to him.

"I guess so. Right here." I confirmed pointing to the itinerary.

During his therapy session, just before my departure for Vietnam, Michael had a request. He wouldn't be traveling back there with our party. But he was hoping to make the pilgrimage in spirit with some help. Only it came across as polite and unassuming as I had come to anticipate from a humble, respectful man like him.

"I have something I want to show you," he said as he pulled his smart-phone from his pocket and accessed his photos.

Michael displayed the two instamatic images he wished to accompany me on my journey to the place where he lost his youth. One was the battered face of the soccer stadium in Bến Tre. The untamed vines already began wrapping themselves around the portico to reclaim what the hands of men had carved out of the jungle.

The other picture depicted the Viet youth and smiling American soldier whose paths crossed so long ago in that Mê Kông Delta town. The playful seven-year-old boy affectionately rested on the GI's shoulder. The incongruous pair posed on the steps of the battle-scarred stone facade of the old soccer stadium. During the Tet Offensive of 1968, it served as cover for the surprised South Vietnamese forces as enemy guerrillas turned their fury on the stunned defenders. It's once ornate, pock-marked walls testified to the better days that faded ever since war returned to Bến Tre.

I sat, my eyes locked on that smiling teenager in the picture who now sat in my office, bearing a faint resemblance to the grainy image. I was going to the town in which that photograph was taken five decades earlier. Though Michael wouldn't have imposed, if that stadium still stood, I knew I needed to find it. And in that moment, this became an important way-point in my broader mission.

I chose to go to Vietnam for many reasons. I needed to walk the land, ride the rivers, and explore the jungles in which so many of my veterans lost so much. I wanted to feel the country about which I heard countless stories. I needed to look our former enemy in the face and see what lay behind those eyes. Finally, I wanted to create experiences of a peaceful Vietnam for myself that sat alongside the countless stories of combat in my head.

Over twenty-six years of stories. Stories of fear, horror, loss, death, and destruction. Inextricably laced among those were also countless tales of courage, sacrifice, hope, resilience, patriotism, dedication and love. I needed to make sense of this distant country which lived in my mind trapped in a perpetual state of war.

And because of that, I wanted to find the place where a young soldier found a moment to smile in the midst of his hell. I had to find it for him. I had to find it for me.

During the war, Bến Tre was the seat of the National Liberation Front (NLF), whose political and counterinsurgency movement became better known as the VC. The Vietnamese government erected a museum in honor of those guerrilla fighters who took the battle to the Americans and ultimately won their country back.

That's why we were going to Bến Tre.

Accompanying us on this trek was Tầm Tiền. He hosted our travel group at his island hostel on the north side of the Mê Kông River. He became a dear friend of the leaders of Soldier's Heart and, as a VC infantry captain during the war, was our former enemy. Though every annual travel itinerary to Vietnam this organization sponsored was unique based on the healing needs of the returning veterans, a stay with Tầm Tiền became a staple.

One of the combat veterans in our travel group served as a field grade Army infantry officer with First Aviation in 1968. He, too, had a mission on this leg of the trip. During the war, his best friend was killed at Vĩnh Long Airfield. This was also why we were heading south into the Delta. Just across the Mê Kông River from Tầm Tiền's hostel lay the town of Vĩnh Long.

Upon learning where we would spend the next two nights, the former First Lieutenant's response was just like his personality—curt and to the point.

"Fuck that. I'm not staying with a VC on an island."

The jarring intersection of itinerary details and his trauma history was too much for him to absorb. On the second day of that stay, we planned to cross the river by ferry into Vĩnh Long to pay homage to his fallen friend. Somehow, staying with his former enemy within mere miles of that former American airfield felt like sacrilege.

The group challenged the Lieutenant's refusal. We asked him to lean into his pain so that he might find the healing he waited fifty years and travelled 8,300 miles to find. He reluctantly agreed to come with us to stay with his former antagonist.

After our boat docked on the island, Tầm Tiền came down to the decaying concrete moorings to greet our party. He donned pink-striped pajamas and supported his stout, crooked frame with his cane. He hobbled to the edge of the gangway bearing a cheek-splitting smile.

Our native guide, interpreter, and former ARVN Air Force officer during the war, Trần Đĩnh Sống (Sống), greeted our joyful island host. He announced to our group that Tầm Tiền apologized for greeting his guests in his PJs, adding that he had felt ill lately. He quickly exchanged another few sentences before Sống turned to our group to translate.

"He says that he was not feeling well but knowing his American friends were coming cured him. He says he feels so much better now that you all are here with him!"

With that, Tầm Tiền cheerfully greeted and hugged every guest, friend and stranger alike. Our reluctant Lieutenant, who eventually agreed to stay on the island, visibly stiffened.

One by one, the line of guests patiently moved through the hostel's front gate. Tầm Tiền's affectionate greeting inched closer to the wary veteran before he surrendered to the unavoidable embrace of his former foe.

Later, that night, after a celebratory feast prepared by Tầm Tiền's family, we sat around the long dining table in the bamboo and palm leaf

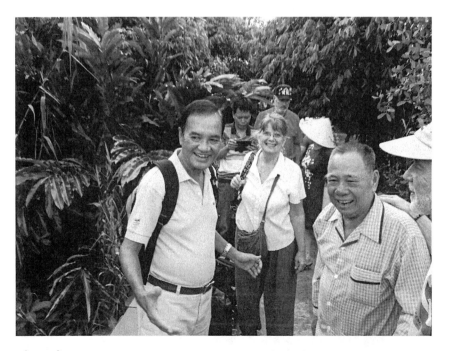

Tầm Tiền, former Viet Cong Captain, greets our Soldier's Heart party at his island boat ramp: Left to right: Trần Đĩnh Sống ("Sống," our guide), Colonel (R) Đặng Vương Hưng (poet and former NVA soldier), Kate Dahlstedt, Michael Snyder (friend of author), unknown (conical hat), Tầm Tiền and Dr. Edward Tick.

shrouded outdoor platform patio. The humid night air carried the rhythmic ballad of the tree frogs surrounding us. A long, magical evening of connection and healing ensued.

After the meal, Tầm Tiền positioned himself proudly at the head of the expansive table of American guests. He summoned one of his children to fetch his mandolin and played a few songs. Though we could not understand the lyrics, we didn't need to; they immediately touched the current of raw emotion beneath the words. Upon the final strum guiding the mournful tales, Sống narrated the euphonious stories.

They were songs of war, and the common burden and pain of men fighting for their lives and their countries. It didn't matter what country. It didn't matter what language they spoke or flag they honored. They expressed the universal plight of warriors that only they could know.

The veterans of our group digested these deeply resonant lyrics and leaned in a little closer. This former VC captain was not who or what they expected.

They cautiously found their way towards one another. Some of them compared their physical war scars in a macabre, well-humored exchange. Tầm Tiền went first.

During one engagement with the Americans, he was shot multiple times and left for dead on the battlefield. He lifted his shirt and displayed the deep craters where he took two 5.56mm rounds through his belly. The third bullet left a jagged, lightly colored dimple where the round exited and claimed a chunk of his left forearm. Because of its massive tissue destruction, Tầm Tiền and his cadres nicknamed this newly deployed, high-velocity M16 ammunition "the poison bullet."

With incredible serendipity, an interpreter-mediated conversation between Tầm Tiền and another American veteran

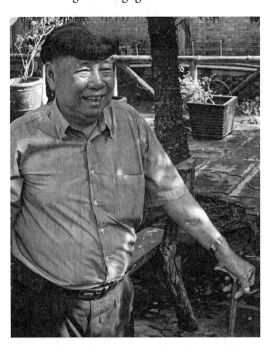

Tầm Tiền's war-wounded forearm.

revealed they fought in the very same battle on the Plain of Reeds in late September of 1968. They sat in stunned silence for a moment, gazes fixed upon one another.

Upon learning of this revelation, Sống smiled after listening to Tầm Tiền's thoughtful response to his foe of a bygone era. He gently turned towards the VC captain's speechless American counterpart.

"He says, I am grateful that we both were bad shots during the battle so we could meet all of these years later as friends."

Two former enemies exchanged smiles of reverence and respect, meeting precisely in the middle of what appeared, only hours earlier, an infinite divide. The tense gap between former enemies continued to melt. Two scarred warriors sat astride, gradually finding their way further into connection.

It was a miraculous scene to witness. I sat in muted awe and turned my attention inward. I recalled the wisdom imparted to me by another combat veteran who overcame his burning hatred of his former enemy. Still fresh, he shared it with me only weeks before my journey to Vietnam. The veteran's words were so profound, they were implanted verbatim, and I vowed to never forget them:

"When you get to hating someone, spend some time with them and you will end up fixing in yourself what you were trying to fix in them."

Another shift in the festivities brought me back to this sacred communal dining table. Tầm Tiền summoned one of his daughters and with a loving smile, offered her some brief instructions, and a nod of assurance to punctuate his request.

Sống turned to the group and began narrating the history of the rare treat we were about to experience. As he continued speaking to the table lined with his guests, the young woman returned carefully cradling a gallon sized mason jar full of a yellow cloudy liquid. Tầm Tiền greeted its arrival with an approving, toothy smile as if the sommelier had just returned with the house's finest.

In the jar, partially visible through the hazy contents, were reptilian features: a webbed foot pressed against the glass, the outline of a spade-shaped head, and the elongated shading of several lizard-like bodies. The lid was sealed with several wrappings of old tape which Sống began carefully removing. As he did so, he continued to tell the story behind its contents.

The jar contained six large, very dead geckos. But these were not just any geckos. Tầm Tiền had paid a million dong ($47) apiece before plunging them into the mason jar of rice wine—a tidy sum for an aging warrior surviving off a small military service pension. They were expensive because Vietnamese tradition believed that the serpents drowned in rice wine imparted medicinal and spiritual healing properties. The jar slumbered for twenty years waiting for an occasion special enough to break the seal.

Tonight was that occasion. We sat, transfixed.

Though I tried cobra snake wine for the first time earlier that day, this felt several steps further into the exotic world of Vietnamese food and spirits; somehow, to my western sensibilities, even poisonous snakes seemed less offensive than large geckos. It didn't matter—I was out of time to think about it. Another daughter suddenly appeared at the table with a small ladle and a tray full of clean shot glasses.

Tầm Tiền beamed with pride as Sống explained the story behind the amber elixir he was now carefully ladling into the shot glasses. The guests near the head of the table gingerly passed the full glasses down the row, one at a time. The heady aroma diffused into the warm evening air.

We sat for hours late into the thick Delta night, talking, sharing, learning, and changing. Whatever hesitancy accompanied the first shot glass of gecko wine began to disappear as the jar's level of golden liquor continued to drop. The conversation yielded to the veterans on both sides, the rest of us circling them in support, intense curiosity, and awe.

Like archetypal warriors sharing stories around a tribal fire, these men talked about their wartime experiences. They compared notes, exchanged critiques of battlefield strategy and tactics, and with each exchange, dug a little bit deeper. By the end of the night, I felt not a single jagged edge between these former foes. The contagion of Tầm Tiền's smile, with the help of some special gecko wine, had done its work. There were many smiles around the table that night.

The following morning, with Tầm Tiền in tow,

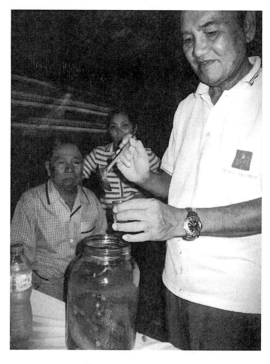

Our guide, Sống, ladles gecko wine at Tầm Tiền's outdoor dining area for his Soldier's Heart guests.

we boarded a small bus destined for Bến Tre. As he hobbled aboard, the grimace of aging bones gave way to his infectious smile. He said something in his native tongue, but our guide and interpreter had not yet boarded.

It did not matter. His joy radiated throughout the cabin. Tầm Tiền, we were told earlier, was on his own mission.

The trip from Vĩnh Long to Bến Tre was only eighty-one kilometers. Because it was the birthplace of the NLF, under whose flag Tầm Tiền fought, it housed the country's tribute museum. Though Tầm Tiền lived most of his life on his island, he'd never been to the city or its museum to honor his service and the many who died under his command. It was a momentous day for him.

We were accompanied by some provincial "guides." Their job was to escort us among the several state-constructed monuments and temples we would visit along the way, all of which enshrined and celebrated Vietnam's national heroes in their long struggle for independence.

Though this wasn't pointed out until we later enjoyed some privacy, Tầm Tiền sat outside every one of them. After he hobbled up to a bench out front, I interpreted his actions as those of an achy septuagenarian resting his weary legs in between our packed travel schedule.

Only he was not resting. He was silently protesting.

These state shrines were a sight to behold. The ornate, marble structures were complemented with large, lavish fresh flower arrangements and beautifully manicured landscapes. They stood in jarring contrast to the dilapidated residences surrounding them. Though Tầm Tiền considered himself a patriot, he didn't care for these temples or the exorbitant resources the state spent on erecting and maintaining them.

Sống later explained Tầm Tiền's perspective. He couldn't understand how the state continued unrestrained spending on these unproductive icons while the people continued to struggle in austerity. We learned that while modern Vietnam was continuing to liberalize its culture and economy, criticism of its communist government remained forbidden.

In America, some protest perceived injustice by taking a knee. Tầm Tiền took a bench. There he sat, propping his battle-scarred arms on his cane while patiently waiting for us to complete our tours. There was one state building, however, that he was eager to visit. It was the only one he entered that day.

The bus pulled into the parking lot of a large yellow and white, French colonial style building. The location of the NLF Museum was no accident. The French long ruled Vietnam as part of their Indochinese empire and wore out their welcome with the Vietnamese people long before American combat troops first arrived. The museum was a tribute to the commoners who rose to first defeat the French, and later fought the goliath American

military. Bến Tre was the birthplace of the resistance, and it now triumphantly celebrated victory in the very building representing the seat of foreign imperial power.

Some sharply dressed museum guides met our party at the entrance.
They were gracious, spoke good English, and appeared quite conscious
of putting on a well-orchestrated tour for their American guests. Sống
appeared more reserved and careful around these polished young men.
They were provincial representatives.

He didn't need to say anything. We got the message; this was not a
place to speak with unguarded candor.

We slowly circulated among the exhibits, pausing to listen to our
guide's rehearsed captions. I soon became bored, and found my attention
wandering. It was then I noticed him. Tầm Tiền wasn't paying attention
either. And he had "the look."

It was the look I'd seen in the eyes of too many of my veteran patients
when they went *back*: back to the bullets, the deafening concussions, the
putrid odors, and the screams of the wounded that continued to wake
them in the middle of the night. It was the far-away look of those who
struggled to find their way back to a present that would save them from the
horror of their past.

I watched his eyes go vacant, and then suddenly shift to another glass
case of war artifacts. Whatever footing his darting eyes eventually found
gave way beneath him as each battlefield item on display beckoned him
back. I scanned the room and then quickly made my way back to him. The
rest of the group appeared engaged with the tour and oblivious to Tầm
Tiền's silent journey into the darkness of his own ordeal fifty years earlier.

The guides' voices dimmed as I absorbed this haunted warrior's every
move. He, too, was preoccupied, my voyeurism unnoticed. His eyes moved
methodically among the cased objects of war, registering each before
scrolling back in his mind to the last time he saw them, seemingly in
another world, part of another life. And yet there they were.

His grazing eyes suddenly stopped, as if stunned frozen by a ghost.
He had found something.

I watched as he hobbled up to get a closer look. Steadying himself on
his cane, he placed a hand on the glass and leaned in closer. Suddenly, he
backed up as if sensing he was too close. His lips began to register words,
though no sound followed. He had discovered something personal. Something he never thought he would see again. But there it was.

Mumbled words became sounds, as he pointed to the rectangular
glass enclosure. I weaved through our crowd to see what was capturing his
attention.

Tầm Tiền was pointing to a neglected French Fusil MAS 36 bolt action rifle. Dating to the 1930s, this relic would have found its way to Vietnam after World War II during the waning years of French occupation. Its antique appearance and uniform infestation of surface rust hinted to its long, troubled service life in the jungle and stirred the imagination of its history. Tầm Tiền, however, was pointing to *his* history.

As a younger man growing up in Cà Mau on the southern tip of Vietnam, he had no interest in politics. He was appointed school master of his small village simply because he was the most qualified for the job; he had the good fortune of a sixth-grade education.

Those were rare days of peace in Vietnam. The French's stunning defeat at Điện Biên Phủ in 1954 gave the country a short reprieve from its thousand-year history of near-constant invasion, occupation, and war. The French left. The Americans had not yet arrived. The village thrived in the calm of the eye of the storm.

One day, war came again. In Vietnam, it always did.

While Tầm Tiền was out on business, bombs fell on his village, struck the school, and killed many of the village's children. A female teacher, who later became his wife, narrowly escaped the smoking rubble. That day, Tầm Tiền became political.

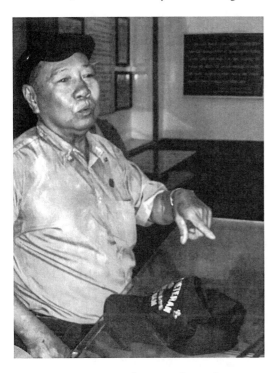

He and this female teacher joined the NLF. They married and took up arms to fight those who had taken their peace. They lived, fought, and gave birth to their young in the jungle. While sharing this story of his past, Tầm Tiền stated his first son, came out "like a coconut."

Sống translated the stark reality of his metaphor. The infant was born severely deformed with an oversized head and under-formed arms and legs and died shortly after birth. Sống explained that Tầm Tiền assumed that bad karma took his first

At NLF museum in Bến Tre, Tầm Tiền points to a World War II-vintage French rifle. He carried one like it during the war.

born away from him. Many years later, he learned this malformation was likely due to the same Agent Orange toxins plaguing American and Vietnamese veterans and their offspring alike for decades after the war.

I watched Tầm Tiền pointing to the rifle in the museum case. His rapid speech attracted Sống's attention, who came to assist the group of us gathered around to hear the mystery the rifle couldn't tell.

"Ah, Tầm Tiền says this is the rifle he carried during the war. One just like this."

Tầm Tiền, the reluctant warrior who fought after war came to him, carried an antique against the modern weaponry of the most powerful military on the face of the earth. He now smiled upon finding a piece of his history and sharing it with our group.

As Sống explained, his smile wasn't about this weapon of war, but his joy that it was in a display case where it belonged, and that he rediscovered it in peace with his American friends. After Sống completed the translation and saw our reactions to his statement, Tầm Tiền's toothy smile widened.

I looked Tầm Tiền in the eye and saw a bright light replace "the look." I didn't need to speak his language to hear what was in his heart. I could see it—his mission had been fulfilled. I looked at the joy in his face and the sense of closure that I wanted to feel. Tầm Tiền's pilgrimage was complete.

Earlier that day, upon sharing the war photograph of the soccer stadium of Bến Tre, and the Vietnamese boy draped over the young American soldier, Dr. Ed Tick and his wife Kate Dahlstedt, our Soldier's Heart group leaders, graciously agreed to add my mission of "return" to the soccer stadium to our busy day trip.

I was too distracted with Tầm Tiền's mission

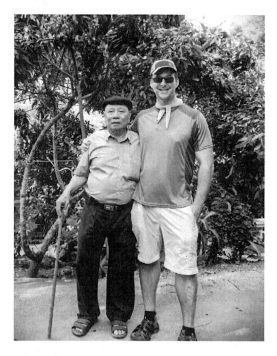

Tầm Tiền and the author on their day of "personal missions" in Bến Tre.

to think of my own. But mine was next on the itinerary. My nervous smile invited his affectionate pat on my shoulder. Because of the language barrier, not a word passed between us. It didn't need to. My heart began to pound. As the tour continued towards completion, I stepped outside for some air.

As I walked outside the museum, I could feel the emotion rising from my gut. I wasn't sure what the message was, but looked for a quiet place to receive whatever was trying to announce itself. I scanned for a spot, and when I saw her sitting alone on a bench outside the museum, I knew I found it.

Kate flashed a kind, inviting smile. I knew I didn't have to ask if I could join her. I sat alongside her and she immediately sensed my need. I had been waiting the entire trip for this feeling to come. The tears came right behind it.

As it washed over me, I began translating its amorphous messages. It started with the present and then continued its descent into my soul. It was about finding the stadium and sitting in the spot where Michael had sat fifty years earlier. It was about my relationships with my veteran patients. It was about making the trip back here that they couldn't, or wouldn't. It was about the thousands of hours I spent with them helping them heal. It was about my dedication to them. No, deeper than that. It was about my love for them.

I don't remember a word Kate said to me that day on the bench. Neither will I ever forget those moments we shared. The world fell away and she simply held it back while I journeyed inward to retrieve the message I needed to understand. A wave of relief spread to every corner of my body.

I watched several veterans in our group take their turns completing their emotional missions of return as we made our way through each carefully planned location. We visited Củ Chi where Ron, an armored truck driver with the 25th Infantry, fought fifty years earlier. We located the exact dip in the road on Route 6 where he survived his first firefight. We completed healing ceremonies for two other veterans: we honored a veteran's best friend who was killed in Vĩnh Long, and constructed another ritual while anchored in the middle of tributary of the Mê Kông River for our "brown water" Navy veteran who served two tours on a patrol boat fighting in those very waterways.

Now it was my turn.

I wasn't a veteran, but my personal mission was taken no less seriously. Ed and Kate assured me we would search for Bến Tre's soccer stadium. However, I hadn't decided what I would do when I found it. Then, as I took my seat on the tour bus, intuition provided the answer. With its arrival, I smiled.

"Of course...," I thought to myself, as my subconscious knew all along and was patiently waiting for the rest of me to catch up.

I anxiously toggled between the pictures Michael gave me, scanning for the stadium's likeness in the structures as they whizzed through the frame of the bus window. Sống motioned the bus driver to stop periodically so he could question the locals for information on its whereabouts. The final time he boarded, I saw the answer in his face.

"David, they said the stadium no longer exists. It was so damaged during the war, they tore it down. A large market is built on the grounds where it once stood."

I was crushed. My anticipation steadily built as I saw several healing missions completed. I saw their relief. I wanted my own. My mind digested the jarring news.

Sống continued, "...but they have a new soccer stadium built at another site. We are only five minutes away. Would you like to...."

"Yes!" I heard myself interrupt before he finished his question.

He smiled and politely shouted some instruction in Vietnamese to the bus driver and within seconds, we pulled back onto the road.

When we arrived, it was not what I envisioned. I silently rearranged the meaning of this return and, with it, followed my intuition which somehow effortlessly filled in the details. In a mere moment, the wispy puzzle completed itself. With it dissolved any traces of any lingering disappointment.

It was perfect.

The Vietnamese had moved on. After centuries of war, they rebuilt their lives and their country. This mission to Vietnam beckoned my veterans and I to do the same. I did not return to a ruin of war. I returned to a place of sport, civil competition, and community gathering in a country now at peace. Vietnam now invited us Americans to move forward with it.

The bus stopped in front of the red marble facade. It was a towering structure and spoke to the country's love of the sport. Its clean, contemporary lines stood in notable contrast to the town's surrounding decrepit structures, with old and new oddly, but comfortably cohabitating.

As planned, Ed followed me out of the bus, my camera in hand. My original plan to recreate the picture with a local youth was upended by the stadium ground's emptiness—there was not a native soul to be found anywhere near the stadium. Now empty and silent, its blank canvas welcomed this foreign visitor to create whatever was necessary. Ed patiently trailed behind waiting for a cue that I found what I needed.

I took one last look at the grainy photo of that teenage soldier, noting his body position, sat on the cool marbled steps, and even without a young accomplice, felt my body align with Michael's.

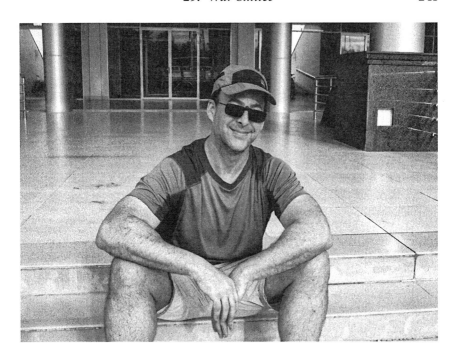

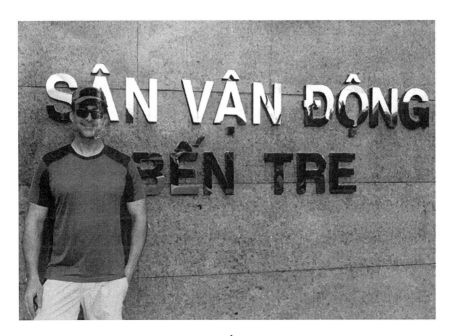

The author at soccer stadium in Bến Tre, 2016 (author's collection).

"Got it!" Ed assured as he smiled upon seeing the glint in my eye. We both took a deep breath in unison. I thanked him with my smile, and he bowed his head and placed his hands together in honor and recognition that another person had done his healing work. He affectionately patted my shoulder as I reboarded the bus. I was greeted with the warm smiles of Tầm Tiền and our veterans. Another mission was complete.

⌒

I studied his face as I handed him the white envelope. He hesitatingly reached for it, silently asking the question of its contents with his raised eyebrows.

I nodded, urging him to open it.

Michael cautiously broke the seal and slid out the contents. I watched his eyes subtly shift to take in the entirety of the two printed images.

The lines of gold lettering in Vietnamese behind me contained the only two words he recognized, but were all that were necessary to translate the meaning of what he was looking at. It was the name of the town in which he had served with the 15th combat engineers so long ago.

He looked up at me before he spoke. He didn't have to say what he was about to, because his eyes said it for him. Then, just as it had fifty years ago, that same smile gradually spread across his face.

Conclusion

This book is about the transformative power of journey and of story. It evolved during a period of intense personal and professional reflection. After twenty-six years of doing trauma recovery work with combat veterans, I was trying to understand my own journey—to figure out where I had been, what I had learned, what I was going to do with this knowledge, and where this would lead me for the final chapters of my professional career; indeed, my life. Over the years, my veterans told me in various ways, "you get it." On one level, this book was my effort to figure out what exactly that meant.

But this quest was anchored in the service of a higher order ambition: I was principally writing to address the unfathomable pain and isolation

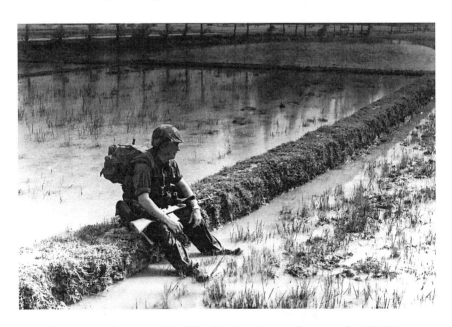

Marine resting on paddy dike, Marine Corps photograph A189962.

243

that veterans suffer because so many others in their lives *don't* "get it" and how I might be of service in bridging that divide. While there is no simple recipe for this, I concluded that others might start learning how to better understand our veterans precisely the way I did—by listening to our warriors' experiences with a sincere heart, opening themselves to what they

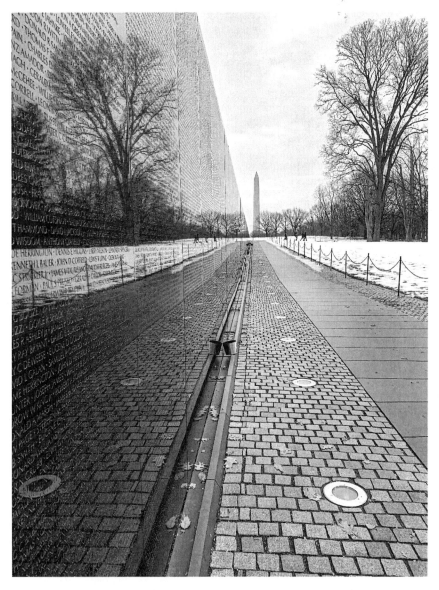

The Wall, Vietnam War Memorial in Washington, D.C. (veteran photograph).

have to teach us, and then transforming during this process. Their stories emerged as that bridge.

While it was obvious that war had forever changed them, what was less evident was that while listening to them, they were transforming me. Throughout history, community transformation, or communalization, was a critical ingredient in healing the traumas of both veterans and those who send them to fight. Somewhere along the way, we lost this ancient wisdom and the practice of including the healing power of community. We have replaced it by relying on experts working behind closed doors to salve the wounded, both of whom then share the immense burden of war in secrecy and isolation.

While we worked hard together to facilitate their healing process, it occurred to me that if these veterans' stories stopped at my office door, something very dear would be tragically lost. Their pain, loss, struggles, triumphs—all of that wisdom, would end at that barrier. With it would die the critical lessons, and deeply deserved understanding and appreciation for their sacrifices they paid on our country's behalf.

Something about this didn't feel right. I felt caught between my professional duty of privacy, and the desire to bridge the divide between our warriors and our community—for all our sakes. I concluded that the best I might do was to share my own journey with you, and with my combat veteran patients' blessings, some of their stories that created it.

However, this journey is not a round-trip ticket. My intent is that upon the completion of this book, like Odysseus' return to Ithaca after the Trojan War, that you too, will in some way, be transformed. And like so many returning combat veterans, you may not recognize the same home you left behind. My hope is that what you discover along the way enriches your life, inspires and engages you in healing our veterans and our community, and provides a deeper appreciation for the gift of your birth rite in our country. For me, it has been well worth the journey.

Glossary

Agency/Spook: Central Intelligence Agency (CIA) field officer.

Agent Orange: the most infamous of the toxic chemical defoliants/herbicides used by U.S. forces to kill vegetation in order to deprive the enemy cover and sanctuary.

Air Medal: awarded for meritorious service while participating in aerial flight. In Vietnam, awarded per twenty-five operational flights during which exposure to the enemy is expected.

AIT: Advanced Individual Training. In the Vietnam era, AIT was typically an eight-week training in one's occupational specialty that followed 8 weeks of basic training.

AK-47: the selective fire 7.62×39mm principal battle rifle for North Vietnamese/VC forces; also known as "Kalashnikov" after its Russian inventor.

AO: Area of Operations. Terrain assigned to specific military units.

APC: Armored Personnel Carrier. Tracked armored vehicle used by mechanized infantry armed with automatic weapons. Also known as "tracks."

Archetype: universal recurring patterns, character symbols, or ideas that represent specific roles or social states that derive from human models or prototypes.

ARCOM: Army Commendation Medal. A decoration presented for sustained acts of meritorious service or heroism; can be awarded with "V device" for valorous actions.

ARVN: Army of the Republic of Vietnam. The armed forces of our allied South Vietnamese government during the war.

Azimuth: a horizontal angular distance or compass bearing from north.

Bird: any military aircraft, but usually referring to a helicopter.

Bivouac: temporary military field encampment in an unsheltered area.

Black Widow: a gun platform of four .50 caliber M2 machine guns mounted on a tracked tank chassis.

Boonies/Bush: slang for being out in the field or jungle on infantry operations; hostile areas outside American firebases or basecamp.

Brown Water (Navy): combat navy forces assigned to internal waterways in Vietnam, usually in the Mê Kông Delta.

C4: plastic explosive carried by combat engineers and infantry. Requires blasting cap or percussion for explosive ignition, but when lit with flame, burns like sterno; can be used to heat C-rations in the field.

C-rations: canned, prepared combat rations with a long-shelf life issued to fielded troops as their daily staple when fresh, packaged, or unprepared foods were unavailable. Surplus rations were regularly issued during the Vietnam War, WWII, and Korean War.

Cache: supply of munitions, usually referring to hidden supplies.

CAP unit: Combined Action Program. A USMC program placing small American combat units in "friendly" villages to fight in coordination with local forces/South Vietnamese militia ("Popular Forces").

CAR15: the shortened, carbine version of the main American battle rifle, the M16. Typically issued to officers or those in recon or special operations.

Charlie: slang for the enemy, specifically Viet Cong (derived from "Victor Charlie" for VC in military radio protocol).

Cherry: slang for a new or inexperienced soldier/replacement in theater.

Chi-com: short for "Chinese Communist" usually in reference to equipment and weaponry.

CIB: Combat Infantry Badge. Awarded to soldiers in the U.S. Army for being under enemy fire in a combat zone.

Civvies: Slang for civilian clothes; out of uniform.

Clacker: M57 firing device, hand-held electric, wire-connected trigger for claymore mines.

Claymore: antipersonnel mine typically deployed by infantry for perimeter defense. Contained C4 plastic explosive and when detonated, propelled 700 steel bearings in a 60-degree fan-shaped cone.

Cloverleafs (Patrol): Connecting circular pattern of infantry foot patrols where the same ground was never covered twice in order to avoid booby traps and ambushes.

Cobra-Bell AH-1 model: the first production American attack helicopter with a two-man crew, and heavily armed with guns and rockets for ground attack role.

Communalization: in trauma recovery specifically, the healing experience of sharing the traumatic narrative with an empathetic and respectful community of peer listeners.

Concertina (wire): razor wire in large, expanding coils used for creating defensive obstacles around fighting positions or perimeters.

Cook-off: slang for something igniting or exploding due to excessive heat.

Corps: geographical division of South Vietnam into four warzones or "Corps" beginning with the most northern ("I Corps") and progressing through II Corps (Central Highlands), III Corps (Sai Gon and Mê Kông Delta region), to the southernmost region (IV Corps).

CP: Command Post

Crew Chief: the helicopter crew member in charge of everything that happens with the aircraft and on board it.

Dear John: slang for a "break-up" letter from a loved one at home to inform the relationship is ending.

DEROS: Date of Expected Return from Overseas. The day marking the end of their combat tour and counted down to with great anticipation.

Det cord: Detonation Cord. Flexible plastic tube filled with explosive that acts as high-speed ignition/fuse for high explosive charges.

Deuce-and-a-half: M35 series standard 2½-ton troop transport/cargo 6x6 truck.

DI: Drill Instructor. Principal instructor for new military recruits undergoing training.

DMZ: the roughly two-kilometer "demilitarized zone" separating North and South Vietnam; the temporary border at the 17th parallel agreed upon at the Geneva Accords in 1954 following the defeat of the French colonists.

Don't mean nuthin': a coping term/mantra coined during the Vietnam War, and used by troops as a way of dismissing and dissociating from witnessing/experiencing something horrific.

Door gunner: combat aircraft crewman/machine gunner positioned at the doors of a combat aircraft, usually a helicopter.

Dress Blues: the issue dress/parade uniform of the United States Marine Corps.

Dress Greens: the issue dress/parade uniform of the United States Army; also, formerly known as "Class A's."

Dust Off: slang for medical evacuation by helicopter.

E-tool: Entrenching tool. Folding shovel carried by infantrymen.

EM Club: Enlisted Men's club/bar on military base for recreation.

FNG: "fucking new guy" or slang for new soldier/replacement in theater.

4F: classification for men deemed unfit for military service usually due to an exclusionary medical condition.

Firebase/Fire Support Base (FSB): temporary artillery encampment used to support forward ground/infantry operations.

Flare: illumination projectile used in night fighting/perimeter defense.

Flechette: small steel dart projectile used in an explosive warhead either fired by artillery, rockets, or by M79 grenade launcher; also known as "beehive" rounds.

Freedom Bird: the airplane returning troops home to the United States after they completed their combat tour (i.e., DEROS'd).

Free fire zone: denotes area of operations cleared of all friendly forces and civilians, thereby assuming all unidentified people remaining to be enemy combatants.

Friendlies: American or allied forces; non-enemy forces.

Friendly fire: accidental casualty caused by weapons fire of one's own armed forces or allies. Formal military term is "misadventure."

GI: Government Issue. Nickname for American troops popularized during World War II.

Grunt: slang for American infantry soldier or Marine.

Gunship: Bell UH-1B "Huey" model helicopter initially pressed into service but too underpowered to carry the extra weight of armament; typically outfitted with fixed machine guns, 2.75-inch rockets, and grenade launchers. UH-1C model subsequently developed specifically for the gunship role.

Gun well: the aft, outwards facing positions in a Huey helicopter where the door gunners were positioned behind their M60 machine guns.

Half-stepping: derogatory slang for being complacent or not paying attention while in the field. A state of combat unreadiness.

Half-track: armored fighting vehicle named for its tank-like tracks on the rear for treaded propulsion, while wheels on the front axle are used for steering.

Ham and motherfuckers: slang for C-ration meal of ham and lima beans.

Hero's journey: the monomyth/archetypal template of stories that involve a hero who leaves the known, enters into the unknown (adventure) to gain something they need, experiences adversity (ordeal) and is tested but ultimately victorious in this decisive crisis, and returns to the known, changed and transformed.

Hỏa Lò: roughly translates into "fiery furnace" in Vietnamese and was the name for the prison built in Hanoi by the French colonial government to hold indigenous political prisoners. Repurposed by the North Vietnamese during the war to hold captured U.S. servicemen, and airmen in particular. Sarcastically dubbed the "Hanoi Hilton" by its American prisoners.

Hot: slang for combat area under fire; typically describing a landing zone.

Huey: nickname for the Bell UH-1 model helicopter, the principal helicopter used in the Vietnam War.

Hump: march or patrol carrying a rucksack in the field.

In Country: slang for being on foreign deployment, in this case, Vietnam.

Jungle boots: standard issue American forces footwear that combined leather and canvas, the latter because it dried quickly and didn't rot as leather would in a tropical, wet climate. They were equipped with drains to aid quick drying and a steel shank for spike protection.

KIA: Killed in Action.

Kill zone: the area within an ambush site or radius around an explosive device where maximum killing/wounding of the target is expected.

Klick: slang for kilometer, or 6/10ths of a mile.

KP: short for "Kitchen Police/Patrol," assigned to kitchen duty.

Laterite: type of soil/rock indigenous to tropical climates that is rich in iron oxide with a characteristic rusty-red color.

LAW: Light Anti-tank Weapon. A shoulder-fired 66mm portable, disposable, fiberglass, single-shot rocket launcher carried by infantry for use against hard targets.

Line company/unit: a combat infantry unit.

Lock and load: loading, arming and readying a weapon by chambering a round.

LRRP: Long-Range Reconnaissance Patrol. A small, elite team of specially trained infantry with a mission of operating deep in enemy territory to observe enemy activity and gather intelligence.

LZ: Landing zone, or clearing used by helicopters to insert combat troops.

M14: the selective fire 7.62mm American main battle rifle in service at the start of the Vietnam War and used for rest of war in more limited capacities.

M16: the selective fire 5.56mm American main battle rifle that replaced the M14 beginning in 1966.

M60: the standard lightweight, belt-fed 7.62mm American machine gun used widely in Vietnam by infantry, armor, and helicopters.

M79: a portable, breech-loaded, single-shot 40mm grenade launcher used by infantry grenadiers; also known as "blooper" or "thumper."

Marston Mat (aka PSP or "perforated steel planking"): interlocking perforated steel panels used for rapid construction of temporary runways.

Medevac: medical evacuation from the field, typically by helicopter.

Mermite (container): U.S. military issue insulated food container.

MIA: Missing in Action.

Mortar: a muzzle-loaded, short-barreled light artillery that launches various size explosive projectiles at high angles. Indirect fire weapon used in close support of infantry operations.

MOS: Military Occupational Specialty, or assigned military job.

Napalm: a jellied gasoline incendiary munition designed to stick to a surface as it burns; typically deployed by air-to-ground bombs but could also be deployed by tank, watercraft, or flamethrower.

NCO: Non-Commissioned Officer. Servicemember usually in charge of a squad or platoon.

NLF: National Liberation Front. The military arm of the South Vietnamese political group who fought as guerrilla fighters in South Vietnam, otherwise known as Viet Cong (VC).

NVA: North Vietnamese Army, or "regulars."

OD: Olive drab. The ubiquitous color of most military field gear, vehicles, and uniforms in the United States military.

Ordnance: military munitions, usually referring to artillery or aircraft munitions.

P38: standard issue tiny, folding can opener used by soldiers to open their C-rations.

Piasters or "Pi": basic Vietnamese monetary unit.

Pith helmet: North Vietnamese infantry issue, lightweight, cloth-covered tropical/sun helmet.

Point: the first/most forward man or element on a combat patrol.

POW: Prisoner of War.

PTSD: Post-Traumatic Stress Disorder is an emotional injury in response to traumatic event(s). While immediate trauma symptoms are expected and often adaptive, this can crystalize into syndrome consisting of psychological, behavioral and moral symptoms and suffering that inhibits recovery.

Punji sticks: sharpened stakes of bamboo or metal buried in ground/pits as a booby trap. Often poisoned with feces to cause infection. Usually arranged in pits on or beside trails and camouflaged.

Purple Heart: decoration awarded by the American military for being wounded or killed (posthumously) by the enemy while engaged in military operations.

PX: Post Exchange. Retail store on a military camp or installation.

Quonset hut: a lightweight, prefabricated, semi-circular/cylindrical military building constructed of corrugated steel.

RA: the prefix for regular army, or volunteer soldiers.

R&R: Rest and Recreation. A short break from the war.

RPG: Rocket-propelled grenade. A shoulder-fired, rocket-motored missile with explosive warhead, made in Russian or China, and used extensively by communist forces.

RTO: Radio/Telephone Operator, or radioman.

Rucksack/Ruck: standard issue infantry backpack.

RVN: Republic of Vietnam.

S2: military organizational structure related to specific duties. S1-Personnel; S2-Intelligence; S3-Training & Operations; S4-Supply & Logistics.

Saddle up: getting combat equipment/rucksack and prepare to move.

Sapper: an enemy commando usually armed primarily with explosives tasked with attacking hard targets.

Satchel charge: pack filled with explosives that is dropped or thrown at enemy positions.

Seabag: standard issue duffle bag.

Semper Fidelis: Latin term meaning "always faithful." The motto of the United States Marine Corps.

Shit can: slang for discarding/disposing of anything unnecessary.

Short: denoting combat tour is almost over. A period of looking forward to going home but usually with more intense fear of not surviving.

Short round: indirect weapons fire (artillery, mortar, etc.) that falls short of its target.

Shrapnel: high-velocity fragments of munition metal casing sent flying by exploding shell.

Sit-rep: Situation report. The regular radio checks provided by field units to the company or battalion radio operators.

Skids: the two parallel metal tubes that make up the landing gear on helicopter.

Slick: Bell UH-1B "Huey" model Helicopter used primarily for troop and supply transport.

Soldier's Heart, Inc.: a nonprofit organization (now closed) founded by Dr. Edward Tick and his partner, Kate Dahlstedt, that was dedicated to transformational work with veterans in healing and restoring emotional, moral, and spiritual wounds of war and military service. Both are now carrying forward that same mission in private practice.

SP: Sundries pack. Accompanied C-ration cases and contained toiletries, cigarettes, and other "luxury" items for fielded troops.

Starlight scope: a light-intensifying scope and early night vision technology that helped to identify targets in the dark.

Steel pot: standard issue U.S. military steel combat helmet.

Tet Offensive: massive, coordinated attacks by North Vietnamese and VC forces on numerous military installations and cities in South Vietnam launched on the Vietnamese New Year ("Tet") on January 31, 1968.

Thousand-yard stare: the vacant/unfocused look of exhaustion/detachment that can result from heavy combat exposure in war-weary soldiers; form of psychological dissociation from trauma/horror.

Tracer: chemically treated small arms cartridge that glowed when fired so its flight path could be followed; American forces typically used red while the Vietnamese typically used green tracers.

U.S.: the prefix for United States troops who were drafted.

USMC: United States Marine Corps.

Utilities (jungle): standard American military issue lightweight, ripstop tropical battle fatigues.

VC: Viet Cong. The communist guerrillas who fought against U.S. troops.

Viet Minh: shortened name for the independence movement organization (League for the Independence of Vietnam) launched by Ho Chi Minh in 1941 to gain independence from France.

Ville: Vietnamese village or hamlet.

Web gear: combat belt and shoulder harness for packing equipment and ammunition on infantry operations.

WIA: Wounded in Action

Wood line: row of trees at the edge of a field, rice paddy, or jungle section.

The World: getting back to "real" life/returning to United States.

Xin loi: Vietnamese idiom for "Sorry about that."

Index

Numbers in **bold italics** indicate pages with illustrations